W0225729

NEW PERSPECTIVES IN HEMODIALYSIS, PERITONEAL DIALYSIS, ARTERIOVENOUS HEMOFILTRATION, AND PLASMAPHERESIS

ADVANCES IN EXPERIMENTAL MEDICINE AND BIOLOGY

Editorial Board:

NATHAN BACK, *State University of New York at Buffalo*

IRUN R. COHEN, *The Weizmann Institute of Science*

DAVID KRITCHEVSKY, *Wistar Institute*

ABEL LAJTHA, *N. S. Kline Institute for Psychiatric Research*

RODOLFO PAOLETTI, *University of Milan*

Recent Volumes in this Series

A Continuation Order Plan is available for this series. A continuation order will bring delivery of each new volume immediately upon publication. Volumes are billed only upon actual shipment. For further information please contact the publisher.

NEW PERSPECTIVES IN HEMODIALYSIS, PERITONEAL DIALYSIS, ARTERIOVENOUS HEMOFILTRATION, AND PLASMAPHERESIS

Edited by

**W. H. Hörl and
P. J. Schollmeyer**

Medizinische Universitätsklinik
Freiburg, Federal Republic of Germany

PLENUM PRESS • NEW YORK AND LONDON

Library of Congress Cataloging in Publication Data

International Symposium on New Perspectives in Hemodialysis, Peritoneal Dialysis, Arteriovenous Hemofiltration, and Plasmapheresis (1988: Freiburg, Germany)
  New perspectives in hemodialysis, peritoneal dialysis, arteriovenous hemofiltration, and plasmapheresis / edited by W. H. Hörl and P. J. Schollmeyer.
    p.   cm. — (Advances in experimental medicine and biology; v. 260)
  Proceedings of an International Symposium on New Perspectives in Hemodialysis, Peritoneal Dialysis, Arteriovenous Hemofiltration, and Plasmapheresis, held October 6-8, 1988, in Freiburg, Federal Republic of Germany" — T.p. verso.
  Includes bibliographical references.

  1. Hemodialysis — Congresses. 2. Peritoneal dialysis — Congresses. 3. Continuous arterio-venous hemofiltration — Congresses. 4. Plasmapheresis — Congresses. I. Hörl, Walter H. II. Schollmeyer, P. J. III. Title. IV. Series.
  [DNLM: 1. Hemodialysis — congresses. 2. Hemofiltration — congresses. 3. Peritoneal Dialysis — congresses. 4. Plasmapheresis — congresses. WJ 378 I5993n]
  RC901.7.H45I575   1988
  617.4'61059 — dc20
  DNLM/DLC   89-22951
  for Library of Congress   CIP

ISBN-13:978-1-4684-5720-9   e-ISBN-13:978-1-4684-5718-6
DOI: 10.1007/978-1-4684-5718-6

Softcover reprint of the hardcover 1st edition 1989

Proceedings of an International Symposium on New Perspectives in
Hemodialysis, Peritoneal Dialysis, Arteriovenous Hemofiltration,
and Plasmapheresis, held October 6-8, 1988, in Freiburg,
Federal Republic of Germany

© 1989 Plenum Press, New York
A Division of Plenum Publishing Corporation
233 Spring Street, New York, N.Y. 10013

All rights reserved

No part of this book may be reproduced, stored in a retrieval system, or transmitted
in any form or by any means, electronic, mechanical, photocopying, microfilming,
recording, or otherwise, without written permission from the Publisher

PREFACE

We are pleased to present our readers the Proceedings of the International Symposium "New Perspectives in Hemodialysis, Peritoneal Dialysis, Arteriovenous Hemofiltration, and Plasmapheresis" which was held in Freiburg i. Br. (FRG) during Octtober 6-8, 1988.

The meeting was held on the occasion of opening the new dialysis unit of the University Hospital of Freiburg i. Br.. The topics discussed included membrane biocompatibility, catabolic factors associated with dialysis therapy, pharmacological therapy in dialyzed patients, erythropoietin and renal anemia, new developments in CAVH, CAPD and plasmapheresis, renal replacement therapy in acute renal failure, and plasmapheresis therapy in systemic diseases. It was unfortunately impossible in this volume, to include the extended, lively and stimulating discussions which were enjoyed by the participants during the conference.

The meeting has provided an unique framework for close interaction between scientists from various disciplines, including nephrology, pharmacology, hematology, cardiology, anesthesiology, surgery, intensive care medicine, and pathology.

We would like to express our gratitude and appreciation for all those who have stimulated, encouraged and supported us to hold the symposium in Freiburg. This endeaver could not have been possible without the generous financial support of Asid-Bonz (Böblingen), Bayer AG (Leverkusen), Bayropharm GmbH (Köln), Baxter (München), Ciba-Geigy (Wehr/Baden), Cilag GmbH (Sulzbach), Fresenius AG (Oberursel), Gambro (Martinsried), Gry-Pharma GmbH (Kirchzarten), Hoechst AG (Frankfurt), Hospal (Nürnberg), Knoll AG (Ludwigshafen), Lederle-Cyanamid (Wolfratshausen), E. Merck (Darmstadt), MSD Sharp and Dohme GmbH (München), Pfizer GmbH (Karlsruhe), and Pfrimmer and Co (Erlangen).

We are indepted to Dr. Jutta Steinbiss, MSD Sharp and Dohme GmbH (München) and Mrs. S. Werth, Hagen GmbH-Kongress-Service for their advice and practical help and to Mrs. I. Szkibik, Mrs. I. Goldbeck, Miss R. Vogel, Miss P. Dämisch for their invaluable assistance and help in the organization of the meeting.

CONTENTS

PROTEIN CATABOLIC FACTORS IN PATIENTS ON RENAL REPLACEMENT THERAPY

Jonas Bergström

Department of Renal Medicine, Huddinge University
Hospital, Karolinska Institute
S-114 86 Huddinge, Sweden

PROTEIN MALNUTRITION IN HAEMODIALYSIS PATIENTS

Several reports have documented that malnutrition is frequently present in patients with maintenance haemodialysis therapy[1-5]. Signs of malnutrition in regular dialysis patients are reduced muscle mass assessed by anthropometric methods, low concentration of albumin, transferrin, and other liver-derived proteins, low alkali-soluble protein in muscle in relation to dry fat-free weight and DNA, abnormal plasma amino acid and intracellular amino acid profiles, similar to those found in untreated uremia, indicating that dialysis does not reverse these abnormalities. It is generally accepted that suboptimal nutritional status is associated with increased morbidity and may contribute to poor rehabilitation and quality of life. Cutaneous energy and other immune alterations strikingly similar to those observed in malnutrition have been documented in haemodialysis patients[3,6,7] suggesting that protein-energy malnutrition may be a risk factor for infection and septicemia. Malnutrition is an important factor for morbidity and mortality in haemodialysis patients[8,9].

PROTEIN AND ENERGY REQUIREMENTS IN HAEMODIALYSIS PATIENTS

Subjects with normal renal function have a minimum daily protein requirement of about 0.5-0.6 g protein/kg/day. Results of nitrogen belance studies in patients on maintenance dialysis twice a week suggested that approximately 0.75 g/kg/day of high biological value protein is necessary to maintain nitrogen equilibrium or a slightly positive nitrogen balance.

According to more recent long-term studies this amount of protein may not, however, be adequate. Signs of malnutrition have been observed in substantial fractions of apparently well-rehabilitated patients on maintenance haemodialysis, who had a daily intake of about 1 g protein/kg body weight/day[1].

HAEMODIALYSIS AS A CATABOLIC STIMULUS

There is evidence that the haemodialysis procedure per se is a strong catabolic stimulus. Borah et al[12] found that during ingestion of a low protein diet (0.5 g/kg BW/day), the nitrogen balance was markedly negative on dialysis days and also slightly negative on nondialysis days. During ingestion of a high protein diet (1.4 g/kg BW/day), the nitrogen balance was still negative on dialysis days, but positive on nondialysis days and the cumulative balance for the study period was not different from 0. It has been found that the urea appearance rate was about 30 % higher during dialysis than off dialysis which confirmed that the dialytic procedure is a catabolic stimulus[13].

LOSS OF AMINO ACIDS

During haemodialysis average losses of free amino acids in the dialysis fluid have been reported to be 5-8 g/dialysis[14,15], of which about one third are essential amino acids. In addition, 4-5 g of peptide-bound amino acids are lost per dialysis[14]; thus, the total losses of amino acids are about 10-13 g/dialysis. Obviously, the losses of free and bound amino acids during dialysis are insufficient to completely account for the increased protein requirements in haemodialysis patients compared to nondialyzed uremic patients. Hence, one may conclude that additional factors not related to the dialytic removal of amino acids (and glucose) are involved.

BLOOD-MEMBRANE INTERACTION

It is now recognized that blood-membrane interaction in a dialyzer induces several biological effects, such as stimulation of the complement system, transient leukopenia, aggregation of granulocytes, and release of granulocyte enzymes, clotting, and thrombocyte activation[16]. These signs of bioincompatibility are especially prominent when using dialyzers with regenerated cellulose (cuprophane) membranes. It has been demonstrated that the blood-membrane interaction induces release of elastase (measured as elastase-α1-proteinase inhibitor complex) and other granulocytic enzymes and it has been speculated on whether such enzymes might have a role in the enhanced catabolism induced by acute uremia and haemodialysis[17]. However, since catabolic granulocyte enzymes, e.g. elastase, are rapidly inactivated in plasma, it is doubtful whether they could have a generalized effect on protein turnover.

More probably, blood-membrane interaction may cause the release of other factors which directly or indirectly induce catabolism of muscle protein.

The interleukin-1 (IL-1) hypothesis links several acute and chronic symptoms in haemodialysis patients to monocyte

2

activation with synthesis and release of IL-1, a family of polypeptides with molecular weights between 17 and 18,000 daltons with a broad range of biological properties associated with both acute and chronic inflammatory changes[18]. Among the effects of IL-1 are fever, leucocytosis, acute phase protein synthesis by the liver, increased muscle protein catabolism, myalgia, tissue inflammation, stimulation of fibroblast activity, induction of collagenase synthesis and bone resorption. IL-1 may act in conjunction with tumor necrosis factor (TNF) or chachexin, another monocyte product, synthetized and released as a consequence of microbial stimulation and tissue injury.

The dialysis membrane may stimulate the generation of IL-1 by a direct effect on adhering monocytes or indirectly by complement activation with release of C5a, which is a known IL-1 inducer. The dialysis fluid is not an innocent bystander considering that acetate used as a buffer source may contribute to IL-1 activation and that endotoxin fragments which are strong activators of IL-1 synthesis and release may pass through the dialysis membranes. We have recently found that sham dialysis (i.e. blood circulation through a dialyzer without circulating dialysate) using cuprophane in non-uremic individuals induces significantly increased muscle protein catabolism (Fig 1)[19], whereas blood-membrane contact with synthetic membranes (PAN, polysulphone) had no such effect[20,21]. The catabolic effect of blood-cuprophane contact could be abolished by pre-treatment with indometacin[19] i.e. was prostaglandin-mediated, being consistent with a role of IL-1, which exerts its protein-catabolic effect in muscle through mediation by prostaglandin E2.

Based on the assumption that the enhanced catabolism induced by blood-cuprophane interaction uniformly involved the total muscle mass estimated to be 40 % of the body weight, the increased release of tyrosine (an amino acid which is not metabolized in muscle) corresponded to an increased protein breakdown of about 20 g. In our experiments on normal man, endotoxin contamination from dialysis fluid was not present and the blood exposure to the membrane was small (blood flow 100 ml/min/m^2 during 150 min) compared with the exposure during clinical dialysis in most haemodialysis patients (higher blood flows, longer times, and sometimes larger surface area). It is thus possible that the stimulating effect on protein catabolism is much higher during clinical dialysis than in our experiments.

ADAPTIVE DECREASE OF PROTEIN INTAKE

It may be difficult to fulfill the requirements of a relatively high protein intake since some haemodialysis patients seem to loose appetite and reduce their protein intake spontaneously, especially if they are underdialyzed with regard to small molecules. Experiences from the National Cooperative Study on Dialysis Prescription[9], conducted in the USA, show that those patients who were dialyzed according to a schedule which implied a low total weekly clearance of urea had a significantly lower urea appearance rate and consequently a lower blood urea nitrogen level than might have been expected if the protein intake had been as high as prescribed.

In conclusion, patients on regular haemodialysis have an increased requirement of protein compared to normal subjects and nondialyzed chronic uremic patients. The enhanced protein requirement is due to (1) loss of amino acids into the dialysis fluid and (2) accelerated protein catabolism with an increased urea appearance rate which is probably induced by blood-dialyzer interaction. If the protein intake is too low to compensate for this enhanced protein catabolism, the patient will suffer from malnutrition, which is one of the most important factors in altered immune function, morbidity, and mortality of haemodialysis patients.

MALNUTRITION IN INTERMITTENT PERITONEAL DIALYSIS PATIENTS

It is common experienced, although rarely communicated in scientific papers, that patients on intermittent peritoneal dialysis frequently show evidence of protein-energy malnutrition and protein wasting[22-24]. Signs of malnutrition, often unrecognized, have been described as the depletion syndrome and are characterized by progressive loss of lean body mass often masked by hydration giving a false impression of stable body weight[22].

LOSS OF PROTEIN AND AMINO ACIDS IN INTERMITTENT PERITONEAL DIALYSIS

Loss of protein in intermittent peritoneal dialysis amounts to about 13 g/10 h[31], but may increase to 38-40 g/10 h or more during peritonitis[25,26] with elevated protein losses persisting for weeks following a period of peritonitis.

Episodes of peritonitis may increase catabolism not only by enhancing protein losses, but also by direct stimulation of protein breakdown, since infection with inflammation is a catabolic stimulus.

CONTINUOUS AMBULATORY PERITONEAL DIALYSIS

CAPD implies that the patients are continuously dialyzed against fluid instilled in the peritoneal cavity which is exchanged 3-5 times per day. This method has now gained widespread acceptance as an alternative to haemodialysis for chronic renal replacement therapy. It is simple, can be handled by the patient himself, and is, therefore, cost effective. CAPD also involves several catabolic factors such as loss of appetite, loss of proteins and amino acids into the peritoneal dialysate, and recurrent peritonitis.

NUTRITIONAL STATUS IN CAPD PATIENTS

A large portion of CAPD patients has signs of subclinical malnutrition, including abnormal anthropometric

4

parameters, low concentrations of plasma, low alkali-soluble protein in muscle, and gradual reduction of total body nitrogen, reflecting a loss of lean body mass and body protein[4,26-29]. Abnormal plasma and muscle free amino acid concentrations are also observed in CAPD patients[30,31]. Only in one study[32] was the plasma amino acid pattern relatively normal.

PROTEIN REQUIREMENTS IN CAPD PATIENTS

Several studies show that nitrogen equilibrium can be maintained, or positive nitrogen balance be achieved during the initial year on CAPD[33-35]. The nitrogen balance has been found to be positively correlated to protein intake[33,35] and to total energy intake[33]. The results indicate that protein intake should exceed 1.0 g/kg/day as an absolute minimum and preferably exceed 1.2 g/kg/day during long-term treatment.

Peritonitits is associated with markedly negative nitrogen balance[1,33] and in patients with a high incidence of peritonitis as well as inadequate nutritional intake anthropometric measurements may show an impairment over time[28].

DECREASING PROTEIN AND ENERGY INTAKE WITH TIME IN CAPD PATIENTS

Nutritional problems may occur in CAPD patients due to a decreased intake of both protein and total energy with time on CAPD[29].

The reduced nutritional intake during CAPD seems to be caused by a decreased appetite, probably due to absorption of dialysate glucose and abdominal distension by the dialysis fluid[37]. Another explanation is that CAPD patients may become underdialyzed. As the total solute clearance falls (due to decrease in residual renal function), the patients may develop uremic symptoms including anorexia with reduced nutritional intake as a consequence.

PROTEIN AND AMINO ACID LOSSES DURING CAPD

Substantial loss of protein into the dialysate is a major drawback with peritoneal dialysis. The reported average loss of protein into the dialysate in CAPD varies between 5 and 15 g in different studies with large interindividual differences. Thus, dialysate protein loss may vary between 20 and 140 g/week in different patients[38].

Protein losses may increase considerably, usually by 50-100% during peritonitis and may remain elevated for several weeks[25,39]. This is mainly due to increased peritoneal permeability. In addition, intraperitoneal sources of dialysate protein may be of importance[38].

Whereas protein losses during CAPD are unparalleled in haemodialysis, the losses of free amino acids into the

dialysate during CAPD are of the same magnitude (per week)
as with haemodialysis or less.

RECURRENT PERITONITIS

One of the most serious complication of CAPD is recurrent peritonitis which in different CAPD programs varies
from one episode in 4-24 months (average value).

Peritonitis is associated with increased losses of
protein in the dialysate by 50-100 % and may remain elevated for several weeks[25,39]. In CAPD patients with mild
peritonitis the dialysate protein losses increased to an
average of 15.1 ± 3.6 g/day[25].

CHRONIC STIMULATION OF PROTEIN CATABOLISM IN CAPD PATIENTS

In addition to low protein and energy intake, protein
and amino acid loss and recurrent peritonitis, there is a
possibility that the dialytic procedure per se increases
protein requirements by stimulating protein catabolism by
substances other than live bacteria. These substances could
be microbial products (endotoxins), acetate, plastics,
silicon, glucose, or other products from the system which
elute into the peritoneal cavity.

In conclusion CAPD patients similar to haemodialysis
patients have more than twice higher requirements of protein
compared to normal subjects and nondialyzed uremic patients.
Factors which may impair protein utilization and enhance net
protein catabolism in CAPD patients are low protein and
energy intake due to adverse effects on appetite associated
with low efficiency of small molecule removal, glucose
uptake from the dialysis fluid, and distenion of the
abdominal cavity. Protein and amino acid losses and enhanced
catabolism of protein induced by intermittent peritonitis
contribute to increased protein requirements in CAPD
patients.

ACKNOWLEDGEMENTS

I am indebted to Drs. Anders Alvestrand, Alberto
Gutierrez and Bengt Lindholm for their support in preparing
the manuscript.

REFERENCES

1.   Schaeffer, G., Heinze, V., Jontofsohn, R., Katz, N.,
     Rippich, T.H., Schäfer, B., Südhoff, A., Zimmermann,
     W., Kluthe, R.:Amino acid and protein intake in RDT
     patients. A nutritional and biochemical analysis. Clin.
     Nephrol. 3:228 (1975).
2.   Delaporte, C., Bergström, J., Broyer, M.:Variations in
     muscle cell protein of severely uremic children.
     Kidney Int. 10:239 (1976).
3.   Bansal, V.K., Popli, S., Pickering, J., Ing, T.S.,
     Vertuno, L.L., Hano, J.E.: Protein-caloric malnutri-

tion and cutaneous energy in hemodialysis maintained patients. <u>Am. J. Clin. Nutr.</u> 33:1608 (1980).

4. Guarnieri, G., Toigo, G., Situlin, R., Faccini, L., Coli, U., Lanini, S., Bazzato,G., Dardi, F., Campanacci, L.: Muscle biopsy studies in chronically uremic patients: evidence for malnutrition. <u>Kidney Int.</u> 24 (suppl 16):S-187 (1983).

5. Alvestrand, A., Fürst, P., Bergström, J.: Intracellular amino acids in uremia. <u>Kidney Int.</u> 24 (suppl 16): S-9 (1983).

6. Mattern, W.D., Hak, L.J., Lamanna, R.W., Teasley K.M., Laffell, M.S.: Malnutrition, altered immune function, and the risk of infection in maintenance hemodialysis patients. <u>Am. J. Kidney Dis.</u> 1:206 (1982).

7. Sengar, D.P.S., Rashid, A., Harris, J.F.: In vitro cellular immunity and in vivo delayed hypersensitivity in uremic patients maintained on hemodialysis. <u>Int. Archs. Allergy Appl. Immun.</u> 47:829 (1974).

8. Degoulet, P., Legrain, M., Reach, I., Aime, F., Devries, C., Rojas, P., Jacobs, C.: Mortality risk factors in patients treated by chronic hemodialysis. <u>Nephron</u> 31:103 (1982).

9. Schoenfeld, P.Y., Henry, R.R., Laird, N.M., Roxe, D.M.: Assessment of nutritional status of the National Cooperative Dialysis Study Population. <u>Kidney Int.</u> 23 (suppl 13):S-80 (1983).

10. Ginn, H.E., Frost, A., Lacy, W.W.: Nitrogen balance in hemodialysis patients. <u>Am. J. Clin. Nutr.</u> 21:385 (1968).

11. Kopple, J.D., Shinaberger, J.H., Coburn, J.W., Sorensen, M.K., Rubini, M.E.: Optimal dietary protein treatment during chronic hemodialysis. <u>Trans. Am. Soc. Artif. Int. Org.</u> 15:302 (1969).

12. Borah, M.F., Schoenfeld, P.Y., Gotch, F.A., Sargent, J.A., Wolfson, M., Humphreys, M.H.: Nitrogen balance during intermittent dialysis therapy of uremia. <u>Kidney Int.</u> 14:491 (1978).

13. Ward, R.A., Shirlow, M.J., Hayes, J.M., Chapman,G.V., Farrell, P.C.: Protein catabolism during hemodialysis. <u>Am. J. Clin. Nutr.</u> 32:2443 (1979).

14. Kopple, J.D., Swenseid, M.E., Shinaberger, J.H., Umezawa, C.Y.: The free and bound amino acids removed by hemodialysis. <u>Trans. Am. Soc. Artif. Int. Organs.</u> 19:309 (1973).

15. Ono, K., Sasaki, T., Waki, Y.: Glucose in the dialysate does not reduce the free amino acid loss during routine hemodialysis of non-fasting patients. <u>Clin. Nephrol.</u> 21:106 (1984).

16. Dorson, W.Jr., Ogden, D.: Special symposium on white cells and complement problems in artificial organs. <u>ASAIO J.</u> 7:41 (1984).

17. Hörl, W.H., Jochum, M., Heidland, A., Fritz, H.: Release of granulocyte proteinases during hemodialysis. <u>Am. J. Nephrol.</u> 3:213 (1983).

18. Dinarello, C.A.: Interleukin-1 - Its multiple biological effects and its association with hemodialysis. <u>Blood Purif.</u> 6:164 (1988).

19. Bergström, J., Alvestrand, A., Gutierrez, A.: Acute and chronic metabolic effects of hemodialysis. <u>Proc.</u>

Int. Symp., Trondheim, p. 254 (Karger, Basel, 1986).

20. Alvestrand, A., Gutierrez, A., Wahren, J., Bergström, J.: Protein catabolism in sham-hemodialysis (S-HD): The effect of membranes with different biochemical properties. Clin. Nutr. 6 (suppl 1):10 (1987).

21. Gutierrez, A., Alvestrand, A., Bergström, J.: Effect of in vivo contact between blood and polyacrylonitrile membranes on leg amino acid exchange in normal man. Blood Purif. 6:365 (1988).

22. Palmer, R.A., Newell, J.E., Gray, E.S., Quinton, W.E.: Treatment of chronic renal failure by prolonged peritoneal dialysis. New Engl. J. Med. 274:248 (1966).

23. Blumenkrantz, M.J., Salusky, I.B., Schmidt, R.W.: Managing the nutritional concerns of the patient undergoing peritoneal dialysis. In: Nolph, K.D. (ed.) Peritoneal Dialysis, p. 345 (Nijhoff, Boston, 1985).

24. Khanna, R., Oreopoulos, D.G.: Complications of peritoneal dialysis other than peritonitis. In: Nolph, K.D. (ed.) Peritoneal Dialysis, p. 441 (Nijhoff, Boston, 1985)

25. Blumenkrantz, M.J., Gahl, G.M., Kopple, J.D., Kamdar, A.V., Jones, M.R., Kessel, M., Coburn, J.W.: Protein losses during peritoneal dialysis. Kidney Int. 19: 593 (1981).

26. Strauch, M., Waltzer, P., Henning, G.E., Poettger, G., Christ, H.: Factors influencing protein loss during peritoneal dialysis. Trans. Am. Soc. Artif. Int. Org. 13:172 (1967).

27. McNeil, K., Siccion, Z., Oreopoulos, D.G.: Nutritional status of patients on long-term CAPD. Peritoneal Dial. Bull. 5:12 (1985).

28. Ray, R., Bower, J.D.: Evaluation of continuous ambulatory peritoneal dialysis. Am. J. Kidney Dis. 3:199 (1983).

29. Williams, P., Kay, R., Harrison, J., McNeil, K., Pettit, J., Kelman, B., Mendez, M., Klein, M., Ogilvie, R., Khanna, R., Carmichael, D., Oreopoulos, D.G.: Nutritional and anthropometric assessment of patients on CAPD over one year: contrasting changes in total body nitrogen and potassium. Peritoneal Dial. Bull. 1:82 (1981).

30. Panzetta, G., Guerra, U., D'Angelo, A., Sandrini, S., Terzi, A., Oldrizzi, L., Maiorca, R.: Body composition and nutritional status in patients on continuous ambulatory peritoneal dialysis (CAPD). Clin. Nephrol. 23:18 (1985).

31. Bergström, J., Lindholm, B., Alvestrand, A., Hultman, E.: Muscle composition in CAPD patients. In: La Greca, G. (ed.) Proc. 2nd Int. Course on Peritoneal Dialysis (Wichtig Editore, Milan, 1985).

32. Dombros, N., Oren, A., Marliss, E.B., Andaerson, G.H., Stein, A.N., Khanna, R., Petit, J.H., Brandes, L., Rodella, H., Leibel, B.S., Oreopoulos, D.: Plasma amino acid profiles and amino acid losses in patients undergoing CAPD. Peritoneal Dial. Bull. 2:27 (1982).

33. Kopple, J.D., Blumenkrantz, M.J., Jones, M.R., Moran, J.K., Coburn, J.W.: Plasma amino acid levels and amino acid losses during continuous ambulatory peritoneal dialysis. Am. J. Clin. Nutr. 36:395 (1982).

34. Lindholm, B., Alvestrand, A., Fürst, P., Tranaeus,

A., Bergström, J.: Efficacy and clinical experience of CAPD - Stockholm, Sweden. In: Atkins, R.C., Thomson, N.M., Farrell, P.C. (eds.) Peritoneal Dialysis, p. 147 (Churchill Livingstone, Edinburgh 1981).

35. Giordano, C., De Santo, N.G., Pluvio, M., Di Leo, V.A., Capodicasa, G., Cirillo, D., Espositio, R., Damino, M.: Protein requirement of patients on CAPD: a study on nitrogen balance. Int. J. Artif. Org. 3:11 (1980).

36. Blumenkrantz, M.J., Kopple, J.D., Moran, J.K., Coburn, J.W.: Metabolic balance studies and dietary protein requirements in patients undergoing continuous ambulatory peritoneal dialysis. Kidney Int. 21: 849 (1982).

37. Von Baeyer, H., Gahl, G.M., Riedinger, H., Borowzak, R., Avderdunk, R., Schurig, R., Kessel, M.: Adaption of CAPD patients to the continuous peritoneal energy uptake. Kidney Int. 23:29 (1983).

38. Dulaney, J.T., Hatch, F.E.: Peritoneal dialysis and loss of proteins: a review. Kidney Int. 26:253 (1984).

39. Raja, R.M., Kramer, M.S., Barber, K.: Solute transport and ultrafiltration during peritonitis in CAPD patients. Am. Soc. Artif. Org. J. 7:8 (1984).

β2 MICROGLOBULIN-DERIVED AMYLOID IN DIALYSIS PATIENTS

E. Ritz, R. Deppisch, and G. Stein

Department Internal Medicine, Ruperto-Carola-
University Heidelberg, and
Klinik für Innere Medizin, Friedrich Schiller-
Universität Jena

In the recent past, a whole spectrum of osteoarticular problems has been recognized in patients on longterm hemodialysis. After the recognition by Assenat et al. (1) of amyloid-related carpal tunnel syndrome in hemodialysis patients whose primary renal disease had not been amyloidosis, many reports confirmed its high prevalence in dialysis patients (2). In addition, joint pain, joint swelling and recurrent hemarthros were recognized as the consequence of synovial amyloid deposits (3) which had many similarities with articular amyloidosis of the AL type (4). Finally, amyloid containing bone cysts, pathological fractures (5) and destructive arthropathy in the appendicular or axial skeleton (6) were noted with increasing frequency. Todate, this new form of amyloid has not been demonstrated in non-dialysed uremic patients. However, in patients with preterminal renal failure, similar amyloid has been recognized as a structural component of matrix stones either within the kidney or passed into the urine (7,8). While extrarenal amyloid, todate, has only been demonstrated in patients on renal replacement therapy, i. e. hemodialysis, hemofiltration or CAPD (9), it is unknown whether the phenomenon is causally related to these treatment modalities or whether it merely reflects longer patients survival and continued exposure to risk. It came as a major breakthrough when such amyloid could be characterized at the molecular level by Gejyo(10). He documented that these amyloid fibrils are derived from the circulating precursor molecule beta-2-microglobulin (β_2m). The clinical problems of dialysis-related amyloid have been reviewed extensively elsewhere (9, 11). This communication will mainly discuss problems of pathogenesis and treatment.

1. The β_2m molecule

As shown in fig. 1, β_2 microglobulin is the light chain of class I major histocompatibility protein antigen (MHC-I). It is composed of 100 amino acids and has a relative molecular mass of 11,700 Dalton. With respect to amino acid sequence and conformation, striking homologies exist with the immunoglobulin L-chain, the precursor of another form of amyloid (AL-amyloid).

Analysis of the three dimensional structure of β_2m indicates that more than 50 % of the molecular is in beta pleated sheet conformation, i. e. the conformation exhibited by amyloid fibrils (12). β_2m is localized exterior to the plasma membrane without being covalently attached to the HLA class I molecule. Consequently, membrane β_2m can exchange with circulating β_2m (13). Cell lines of different origin synthesize and secrete free β_2m, suggesting imbalance of synthesis of the two HLA antigen subunits (14), similar to the known disproportionate synthesis of light and heavy immunoglobulin chains. Expression of MHC class I antigens, and in parallel of β_2m, can be induced by numerous signals, e. g. alpha- and gamma-interferon, mitogens, antigens, growth factors or endotoxin (15,16). Stimulation by antigens and cellular growth factors may explain why plasma β_2m concentrations are elevated in patients with chronic bacterial infections, rheumatological diseases or immuno-regulatory disturbances, e. g. SLE or AIDS, and in malignancies. The main source of circulating β_2m has commonly been thought to be the cells of the immune system, but recent evidence showed that β_2m is a true secretory protein of hepatocytes, the synthesis of which is modulated by IFN but not by IL-1 (17), as demonstrated on the protein and RNA level. As expected from its molecular weight, β_2m is distributed in the extracellular space (18) and cleared by glomerular filtration (19,20). Consequently, in patients with reduced renal function, terminal elimination half life is prolonged (18) and in endstage renal failure plasma levels may be elevated up to 60-fold (19). When human β_2m is injected into nephrectomized rats, extrarenal elimination or biodegradation accounts for less than 3 % of total metabolic clearance (20). It is interesting that after injection of labelled β_2m, tracer uptake by organs in nephrectomized animals parallels their macrophage content - a possible hint as to the site of biodegradation, if this occurs, in the

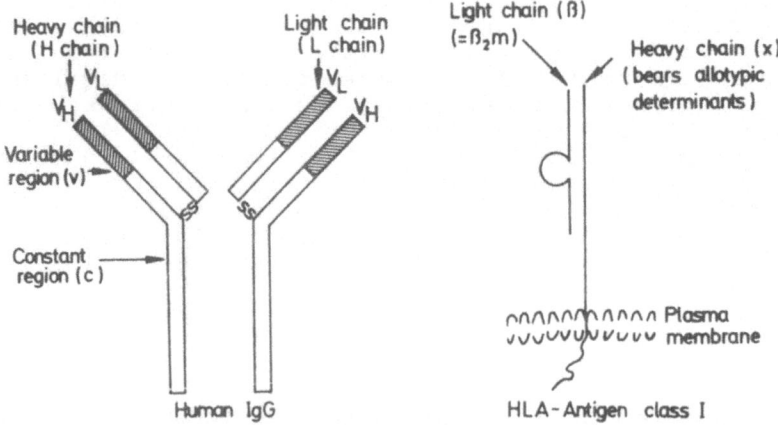

Fig. 1   Schema of molecular structure of IgG and HLA antigen class I.

anephric individual. In dialysis patients, predialysis β_2m levels are importantly influenced by a residual urine volume (21). Normal subjects synthesize (and eliminate via the kidney) an average of 131 µg β_2m/h/kg and similar rates were found in individuals with renal disease (18). More than 95 % of circulating β_2m is monomeric and this is also true in patients with renal failure. A recent communication (22) points to the presence of proteolytically modified "novel" β_2m in dialysis patients, an observation which is of potential relevance to amyloidogenesis. A small, but potentially also important fraction is complex with glyco-proteins, specifically circulating H-chains of the MHC complex (19, 20) or with specific IgG molecules that exhibit strong binding affinity for β_2m (23). Such β_2m containing immune complexes are observed in systemic diseases like sarcoidosis, SLE or PCP. Whether similar immune complex formation is induced by hemodialysis in unknown.

2. β_2m concentrations in dialysed patients

Removal of β_2m across membranes is determined by (i) the molecular cutoff curve of the membrane (ii) membrane structure or morphology and (iii) physicochemistry of the surface involved in blood/membrane interactions. Differen-tial scanning calorimetry showed that homogenous dialysis membranes, e. g. cuprammonium, hemophane or polycarbonate-polyether (24) contain large numbers of pores in the range of 20 Angström. Consequently, significant diffuse or con-vective transport of proteins > 5000 Dalton is impossible. More open high flux membranes, such as polysulfone (F60), hydrophilic polyamide (Polyflux) and polyacrylonitrile (AN 60) permit net removal of β_2m due to their sieving coeffi-cient of 0.6 or better (25). Formation of secondary membra-nes on the surface and/or adsorption of proteins in the microporous structure cause initial increase of the sieving coefficient of β_2m with subsequent decline over treatment time. A hydrophilic modification of polyamide preserves a highly asymmetric membrane structure and also maintains constant sieving characteristics for β_2m (26). When compa-ring β_2m kinetics in different treatment modalities using the same type of membrane, high convective transport in hemofiltration mode reduced β_2m levels 72 ± 18 % (F60) and 62 ± 4 % (Polyflux) respectively, whereas in hemodialysis mode it decreased only by 38 ± 13 and 42 ± 4 % respectively (27). Under these conditions, the total amount of β_2m removed from blood by transport to the membrane and by adsorption can reach 330 mg/treatment depending on pretreat-ment values and exchange volume. In vitro recirculation ex-periments with pooled uremic plasma (28) point to an important role of protein adsorption in removal of β_2m. Mass balance analysis, as carried out by Jorstad et al. (29) is a promising tool to describe transport properties, but is valid only under steady state irreversible conditions.

Acute intervention studies showed lower intradialytic and predialytic β_2m levels when patients were switched from cuprammonium to polysulfone membranes (21,27). Predictably, lower β_2m levels are also found in patients on hemofiltra-tion (30).

In the past, much confusion has arisen from the observation that a marked initial rise, exceeding the increment in hematocrit, is seen in patients dialysed with cuprammonium, but not with polysulfone or PAN membranes. The initial increase of $\beta_2 m$ was interpreted as shedding of $\beta_2 m$ or its fragments from cell membranes in the course of bioincompatibility reactions. Since the space of distribution of $\beta_2 m$ exceeds the plasma volume and is equivalent to the extracellular fluid space (18), it has been suggested that corrections for volume contraction, based on hematocrit only, are inappropriate (31). The conclusion that the mass of $\beta_2 m$ does not acutely change during one dialysis session is inline with the demonstration that during isovolemic dialysis without ultrafiltration or during sham dialysis (blood/membrane contact without dialysis), plasma $\beta_2 m$ levels remain unchanged (32). The failure of $\beta_2 m$ mass to rise acutely does not exclude chronic stimulation of $\beta_2 m$ synthesis by interaction of blood cells with bioincompatible membranes, a possibility which is currently under active investigation in our laboratory.

3. Pathogenesis of $\beta_2 m$ derived amyloid

When analyzed by protein chemistry and immunochemistry (10,33), $\beta_2 m$ amyloid fibrils express $\beta_2 m$ epitopes and show aminoterminal sequence homology with $\beta_2 m$. Molecular weight determinations were reported to show exclusively monomeric $\beta_2 m$ (34). In addition, amyloid fibrils were produced in vitro by salt-free dialysis and concentration of a solution containing intact $\beta_2 m$ polypeptides in the absence of proteolytic treatment (34). It is quite unclear whether comparable conditions ever prevail in the organism.

We (21) and others found no relation between $\beta_2 m$ levels and clinical evidence of $\beta_2 m$ amyloidosis. Passive physicochemical precipitation of $\beta_2 m$ fibrils from monomeric circulating intact precursor polypeptide would also fail to explain a remarkable predilection of amyloid deposition in osteoarticular structures.

We suggested (9,35) and in collaboration with Linke et al. demonstrated (36) that amyloid fibrils consist, at least in part, of proteolytically modified $\beta_2 m$ polypeptides. Amino acid sequence analysis documented truncation of the $\beta_2 m$ molecule at the aminoterminal end, similar to what has previously been described in renal amyloid stones (8) (fig. 2).

```
         1    5      10      15      20     25      30
β₂m   I Q R T P K I Q V Y S R H P A E N G K S N F L N C Y V S G F H P ...
AB₁            I Q V Y S R H P A E N G ...
AB₂                             S N F L N * Y V S G F H P ...
```

Fig. 2 N-terminal amino acid sequence of AB proteins in matrix stones (ref. 8). AB₁ and AB₂ represent $\beta_2 m$-derived amyloid fibril proteins encountered in urinary matrix stones of dialysis patients.

Considerable size heterogeneity on SDS-electrophoresis suggests further truncation at the carboxyterminal end. A consistent feature of proteolytic cleavage was that it occured next to a lysine (or basic amino acid) residue, suggesting action of a trypsin-like protease. The concept of proteolytic removal of a positively charged peptide fragment is inline with the finding of Ogawa (22) who demonstrated "novel" β_2m of lower molecular weight and more acid pI in the plasma of dialysis patients. Limited proteolytic modification is also known to play a key role in the genesis of other types of amyloid causing transformation of the hydrophilic precursor molecule into a more hydrophobic and fibrilogenic product. Proteolytic modification of the β_2m molecule may provide an explanation for the unique pre-ferential localisation of β_2m in osteoarticular structures. Local enrichment of β_2m in articular fluid does not occur as shown by our laboratory and by others (37). This does not exclude, however, local binding of β_2m which interacts with numerous molecules, e. g. with glycoproteins and even with cytomegalovirus envelope (38) presumably because the viral genome codes for a sequence analogous to MCH class I molecules. Based on the scintigraphic finding of increased radiotechnitium uptake in articulations with β_2m amyloid, it has been postulated that low degree local inflammation, e. g. as a result of microcrystaline deposition or hemorrhage, may predispose to amyloid fibril formation (39). Activation of macrophages may be one mechanism involved. Further evidence for a potential role of inflammatory processes may be provided by the finding of Sethis et al. (40) that higher levels of C-reactive protein are found in dialysis patients with as opposed to patients without β_2m derived amyloid.

4. Therapy

Unfortunately, no known procedure is able to reverse existing articular lesions and bone cysts. According to our experience, bone cysts do not regress even after successful transplantation. Anecdotal observations show that pain may respond, although not consistently, to transfer of the patient to more biocompatible membranes or to CAPD. Unfor-tunately, exceptions do occur. Transplantation, although mostly effective in improving pain, does not guarantee a positive outcome. The differential effect of transplantation on pain and on cystic lesions illustrates the important distinction between the active lesion (underlying clinical symptomatology) and the established amyloid deposit (accoun-ting for bone cysts).

Apart from the spectacular efficacy of surgery in carpal tunnel syndrome (9) little can be offered to the patient other than analgesics. However, in patients with pathological fractures, judicious surgical intervention may be indicated. All hope is focused on the development of pro-phylactic measures. In principle, two strategies can be pur-sued. On the one hand, it wil be necessary to develop pro-phylactic measures which permit more effective removal of β_2m. On the other hand, if the above concepts are valid that proteolytic modification, presumably via cellular proteases, is necessary for amyloid fibril formation to occur, pharmacological intervention to inhibit proteolysis may be promising. To draw an analogy: In the prophylaxis of urolithiasis, it is useful to both lower the concentration of the lithogenetic precursor ion and to interfere with nucleation or aggregation.

References

1. Assenat, H., Calemard, E., Charra, B., Laurent, G., Terrat, J.C., Vanel, T.: Hémodialyse, syndrome du canal carpien et substance amyloide. Nouv. Press Méd. 9:1715 (1980).
2. Schwarz, A., Keller, F., Seyfer, S., Poll, W., Molzahn, M., Distler, A.: Carpal tunnel syndrome: a major complication in long-term hemodialysis patients. Clin. Nephrol. 22:133 (1984).
3. Charra, B., Calemard, E., Uzan, M., Terrat, J.C., Vanel, T., Laurent, G.: Carpal tunnel syndrome, shoulder pain and amyloid deposits in longterm haemodialysis patients. Proc. EDTA-ERA 21:291 (1984).
4. Gordon, D.A., Pruzanski, W., Ogrylo, M.A., Little, H.A.: Amyloid arthritis simulating rheumatoid disease in five patients with multiple myeloma. Am. J. Med. 55:142 (1973).
5. Huaux, J.P., Nöel, H., Bastien, P., Malghem, J., Maldague, B., Devogelaer, J.P., Nagant de Deuxchaisnes, C.: Amylose articulaire, facture du col femoral, et hémodialyse périodique chronique. Rev. Rhum. 52:179 (1985).
6. Kuntz, D., Naveau, B., Bardin, T., Drüeke, T., Treves, R., Dryll, A.,: Destructive spondylarthropathy in hemodialyzed patients: a new syndrome. Arthritis Rheum. 27: 369 (1984).
7. Bommer, J., Ritz, E., Tschöpe, W., Waldherr, R., Gebhardt, M.: Urinary matrix calculi consisting of microfibrillar protein in patients on maintenance hemodialysis. Kidney Int. 16:722 (1979).
8. Linke, P.R., Bommer, J., Ritz, E., Waldherr, R., Eulitz, M.: Amyloid kidney stones of uremic patients consist of beta-2-microglobulin fragments. Biochem. Biophys. Res. Commun. 136:665 (1986).
9. Ritz, E., Bommer, J., Zeier, M.: β_2 Mikroglobulinbedingte Amyloidose. Dtsch. Med. Wschr. 113:190 (1988).
10. Gejyo, F., Yamada, T., Odani, S., Nakagawa, Y., Kunimoto, T., Kataoka, H., Suzuki, M., Hirasawa, Y., Shirahama, T., Cohen, A.S., Schmid, K.: A new form of amyloid protein associated with hemodialysis was identified as β_2 microglobulin. Biochem. Biophys. Res. Commun. 129:701 (1985).
11. Van Ypersele de Strihou, C., Honhon, B., Vandenbroucke, J.M., Huaux, J.P., Nöel, H., Maldagüe, B.: L'amylose du dialyse. Actualités Néphrologiques. Flammarion, Paris, 371 (1987).
12. Becker, J.W., Reeke, G.N.: Three dimensional structure of $\beta_2 m$ microglobulin. Proc. Nat. Acad. Sci. (Wash.), 82:4225 (1985).
13. Bernabeu, C., van de Rijn, M., Lerch, P.G., Terhorst, C.P.: β_2 microglobulin from serum associates with MHC

class I antigens on the surface of cultured cells. <u>Nature</u> (Lond.), 308:642 (1984).

14. Evrin, P.E., Nilsson, K.: β_2 microglobulin production in vitro by human hematopoetic mesenchymal and epithelial cells. <u>J. Immunol.</u> 112:137 (1974).

15. Rosa, F., Fellons, M., Dron, M., Tovey, M., Revel, M.: Presence of abnormal β_2 microglobulin in RBA in Daudi cells. Induction by interferon. <u>Immunogenetics</u> 17:125 (1983).

16. Collins, T., Lapierre, L.A., Fiers, W., Strominger, J.L., Pober, J.S.: Recombinant human tumor necrosis factor increases mRNA levels and surface expression of HLA-A, B antigens in vascular endothelial cells and dermal fibroblasts in vitro. <u>Proc. Nat. Acad. Sci.</u> (Wash.) 83:446 (1986).

17. Ramadori, G., Mitsch, A., Rieder, H., Meyer zum Büschenfelde, K.-H.: Alpha- and gamma-interferon (IFN, IFN) but not interleukin-1 (IL-1) modulate synthesis and secretion of β_2-microglobulin by hepatocytes. <u>Eur. J. Clin. Invest.</u> 18:343 (1988).

18. Karlsson, F.A., Groth, T., Sege, K., Wibell, L., Peterson, P.A.: Turnover in humans of β_2 microglobulin: the constant chain of HLA antigens. <u>Eur. J. Clin. Invest.</u> 10:293 (1980).

19. Vincent, C., Revillard, J.P., Gallard, M., Traeger, J.: Serum β_2 microglobulin in hemodialysed patients. <u>Nephron</u> 21:260 (1978).

20. Nguyen-Simonet, H., Vincent, C., Gauthier, C., Revillard, J.P., Pellet, M.V.: Turnover studies of human β_2 microglobulin in the rat. Evidence for a β_2 microglobulin binding plasma protein. <u>Clin. Sci.</u> 62:403 (1982).

21. Bommer, J., Seelig, P., Seelig, R., Geerlings, W., Bommer, G., Ritz, E.: Determinants of plasma β_2m microglobulin concentration. Possible relation to membrane biocompatibility. <u>Nephrol. Dial. Transplant.</u> 2:22 (1987).

22. Ogawa, H., Saito, A., Oda, O., Nakajima, M., Chung, T.G.: Detection of novel β_2-microglobulin in the serum of hemodialysis patients and its amyloidogenic predisposition. <u>Clin. Nephrol.</u> 30:158 (1988).

23. Vincent, C., Revillard, J.P.: Autoantibodies specific for β_2 microglobulin in normal human serum. <u>Molec. Immunol.</u> 20:877 (1983).

24. Göhl, H., Raff, M., Harttig, H., Deppisch, R.: PC-PE-hollow fiber membrane; structure, performance, characteristics and manufacturing. <u>Blood Purif.</u> 4:23 (1986).

25. Flöge, J., Granolleras, C., Göhl, H., Smeby, L., Koch, K.M., Shaldon, S.: Hydrophilic high flux polyamide membranes for beta-2-microglobulin removal. <u>Proc. ASAIO</u>, 10 (1987).

26. Olbricht, C.J., Häbel, U., Frei, U., Koch, K.M.: Effects of runing time on functional characteristics of hemofilters in CAVH. <u>Blood Purif.</u> 5:301 (a) (1987).

27. Flöge, J., Granolleras, C., Koch, K.M., Shaldon, S.: β_2 microglobulin kinetics during hemodialysis and hemofiltration. <u>Nephrol. Dial. Transpl.</u> 1:223 (1987).

28. Goldman, M., Dhaene, M., Vanherweghem, J.L.: Removal of β_2 microglobulin by adsorption on dialysis membranes. <u>Nephrol. Dial. Transpl.</u> 2:576 (1987).

29. Jorstad, S., Smeby, L.C., Balstad, T., Wideroe, T.E.: Removal, generations and adsorption of β2 microglobulin during hemofiltrations with five different membranes. Blood Purif. 6:96 (1988).

30. Kaiser, J., Hagemann, J., v. Herrath, D., Schaefer, K.: Different handling of β2 microglobulin during hemodialysis and hemofiltration. Nephron 48:132 (1988).

31. Bergström, J., Wehle, B.: No change in corrected β2 microglobulin concentration after cuprophane haemodialysis. Lancet I:628 (1987).

32. Bommer, J., Ritz, E., Seres, T., Bommer, G.: Evidence against shedding of β2 microglobulin during hemodialysis with cuprammonium membranes. Arquivos de Medicina 1:316 (1988).

33. Bardin, T., Zingraff, J., Kuntz, D., Drüeke, T.: Dialysis-related amyloidosis. Nephrol. Dial. Transpl. 1:151 (1986).

34. Connors, L.H., Shirahama, T., Skinner, M., Fenves, A., Cohen, A.S.: In vitro formation of amyloid fibrils from intact β2 microglobulin. Biochem. Biophys. Res. Commun. 31:1063 (1985).

35. Ritz, E., Bommer, J., Hänsch, M., Rauterberg, E.W.: Beta-2-microglobulin derived amyloid - unsolved problems and unvertainties about dialytic strategies. VIII é Symposium Gambro: Arthropathies des Dialyses et Amylose B-2 M, Paris (1987).

36. Linke, R., Hampl, H., Lobeck, H., Ritz, E., Waldherr, R., Eulitz, M.: Lysine-specific cleavage of β2 microglobulin in amyloid associated with hemodialysis. Kidney Int. (in press) (1988).

37. Sethi, D., Gower, P.E.: Synovial fluid β2 microglobulin levels in dialysis arthropathy. New Engl. J. Med. 315:1419 (1986).

38. McKeating, J., Griffith, P.D., Grandy, J.: Cytomegalovirus in urine specimens has host β2 microglobulin bound to viral envelope: a mechanism of evading the host immune response? J. Gen. Virol. 68:785 (1987).

39. Sethi, D., Woodrow, D.F., Brown, E.A.: Beta-2-microglobulin derived amyloid and iron in dialysis arthropathies. Nephrol. Dial. Transpl. 2:449 (1987).

40. Sethi, D., Muller, B.R., Brown, E.A., Maini, R.N., Gower, P.E.: C-reactive protein in hemodialysis patients with dialysis arthropathy. Nephrol. Dial. Transpl. 3:269 (1988).

MECHANISMS AND CONSEQUENCES OF COMPLEMENT ACTIVATION

DURING HEMODIALYSIS

Michel D. Kazatchkine and Nicole Haeffner-Cavaillon

Unité d'Immunopathologie, Inserm U28, Hopital Broussais, 96, rue Didot, 75014 Paris, France

Activation of the complement system and secondary leukocyte activation mediate, both directly and indirectly, the acute and chronic effects resulting from immunological bioincompatibility of extracorporeal circuits. This manuscript briefly reviews the mechanisms and consequences of complement activation during hemodialysis. It focuses on recent studies from our laboratory suggesting a role for specific antibodies in the initiation of alternative pathway activation by cellulosic membranes, and indicating that circulating monocytes are stimulated to produce Interleukin-1 (IL-1) _in vivo_ during bioincompatible hemodialysis.

COMPLEMENT ACTIVATION DURING HEMODIALYSIS

Complement activation invariably occurs during hemodialysis with first use cellulosic or Cuprophane hollow fiber dialyzers (Chenoweth et al., 1983a; Hakim et al., 1984). Activation may be quantitated by measuring the plasma concentration of the C3a/C3adesArg antigen in the venous line of the hemodialyzer. During dialysis with Cuprophane membranes, the plasma concentration of C3a antigen rapidly increases during the first 15 min of dialysis to reach 2000-8000 ng/ml, which represents approximately 3 to 10 % cleavage of circulating C3. After 15-20 min, the C3a/C3adesArg antigen concentration decreases and returns to predialysis values at the end of the dialysis session. The decrease in C3a concentration partly reflects the catabolism of the molecule and its transmembrane passage (Smeby et al., 1986). It also reflects a progressive loss in the activating capacity of Cuprophane during the first half hour of dialysis, which is probably secondary to passivation of the membrane with serum proteins rather than to saturation of available C3b-binding sites by covalently bound C3b molecules. Used Cuprophane membranes are coated with C3 fragments which had first been suggested to be ester-linked C3b molecules (Chenoweth, 1984). Recent studies have characterized these fragments as mostly consisting of non-covalently bound C3c (Cheung et al., 1989). Passivation of membranes results in

(Cheung et al., 1989). Passivation of membranes results in decreased complement activation with reused membranes as compared with first-use membranes (Hakim and Lowrie, 1980; Chenoweth et al., 1983b). Complement activation with cellulosic membranes occurs through the alternative pathway as shown by an increase in the plasma concentration of the Ba fragment of Factor B and the lack of significant increase in the concentration of C4a. The rapid rate of C3 cleavage occuring, following the contact of blood with cellulosic membranes is directly related to the high density of sites on the membrane on which bound C3b is relatively protected from H and I and may efficiently interact with Factors B and D to form surface-bound amplification C3 convertase sites (Kazatchkine and Nydegger, 1982). Thus, in an in vitro model, we have shown that C3b bound to Sephadex, a structural analog of Cuprophane, is relatively resistant to inactivation by H and I in whole serum (Carreno et al., 1988a). In addition, the high density of OH-groups that are available for C3b binding on unpassivated membranes, increases the chances for a newly generated C3b molecule to bind in close vicinity of a surface-bound C3 convertase complex in order to form a C5-cleaving enzyme. Thus, the relative efficiency of C5 cleavage relative to that of C3 cleavage on Sephadex is much higher than in the case of other activators such as immune complexes (Bhakdi et al., 1988). This may explain why significant amounts of C5a may be generated upon complement activation in extracorporeal circuits although relatively small amounts of C3 are being cleaved.

The activating capacity of polysaccharides may be influenced by the length of the sugar chain to which C3b has covalently bound (Pangburn, 1987) and by chemical substitution of oligosaccharidic units of the polymer. Substitution of Sephadex with carboxymethylgroups or carboxymethyl sulfonates suppresses the alternative pathway activating capacity of the polysaccharide. The inability of substituted Sephadex to activate complement is due to the formation of stable ternary complexes between H, bound C3b and carboxymethyl groups on the substituted polymer (Carreno et al., 1989). A similar mechanism is likely to be operative in the case of cellulosic membranes on which hydroxyl groups have been modified by addition of a diethylaminoethyl group (Hemophan[R]).

In contrast to cellulosic membranes, polyacrylonitrile and polysulfone membranes induce no or very mild C3a generation. The membranes induce little or no C3 cleavage upon incubation with normal human serum in vitro and adsorb the small amounts of C3a that may have been generated. Rates of C3 cleavage are in any case insufficient to induce the cleavage of C5 and generation of C5a.

An early observation made in patients dialyzed with cellulosic membranes was that the amount of C3a generated could differ considerably between patients dialyzed with the same type of membrane under similar conditions (Hakim et al., 1984). High rates of C3 cleavage were suggested to be associated with an increased risk of occurrence of wheezing, chest tightness and dsypnea ("First-use" syndrome) within the first 30 minutes of dialysis. The serum of patients who amounts of C3a when incubated with Zymosan in vitro (Hakim et al., 1984). Recent studies from our laboratory suggest that differences in the rate of alternative pathway activation by Cuprophane depend on differences in the serum content in anti-dextran antibodies (Weiss et al., 1988). Using Sephadex (1-6 α dextran), we found that although an alternative pathway C3 convertase may be formed on the polymer surface in the presence of purified alternative pathway proteins and in the absence of antibodies, the presence of anti-dextran antibodies greatly enhances alternative pathway-mediated C3 cleavage in whole plasma (Carreno et al., 1988b). Adsorption of normal human serum with Sephadex at 2°C totally suppressed alternative pathway activation in that serum when reexposed to fresh Sephadex particles. Complement activation by Sephadex could be restored in adsorbed serum by coating the polymer with IgG purified from the plasma of a "high responder" individual to Sephadex. The titer of anti 1-4 α dextran antibodies in serum as determined by ELISA was directly related to the extent of alternative pathway activation in whole serum in the presence of Sephadex. The enhancing capacity of IgG antibodies on alternative pathway activation by Sephadex was specific for Sephadex, Fc-independent and analogous to previously observed alternative pathway enhancing antibodies e. g. for Zymosan (Schenkein and Ruddy, 1981) or mouse and rabbit erythrocytes (Moore et al., 1981). In a similar fashion to Sephadex, activation of the alternative pathway in whole serum by Cuprophane in vitro greatly differs in its extent between individuals, and may be totally suppressed by preadsorption of the serum with Cuprophane. A direct relationship exists between the relative capacity of Sephadex and that of Cuprophane to activate the alternative pathway. Although it is as yet unlear whether anti-Sephadex antibodies are similar to anti-Cuprophane antibodies, a direct relationship (r = 0.65) was found between the serum titer of anti-dextran antibodies in the serum of patients dialyzed with Cuprophane membranes and the amount of C3a generated <u>in vivo</u> in the patients at 15 minutes of dialysis. Thus, determining the amount of dextran-reactive antibodies may potentially provide a means of identifying patients at high risk of complement activation with cellulosic membranes.

As mentioned above, alternative pathway activation by polysaccharidic surfaces results in efficient coupling of C5 convertase formation relative to C3 convertase formation and in generation of C5a and C5adesArg. Increased concentrations of C5a/C5adesArg antigen have been found in the plasma of patients dialyzed with Cuprophane membranes. The extent to which C5 ist cleaved <u>in vivo</u> has however been difficult to assess because of transmembrane passage of C5a and high affinity binding to specific receptors on leukocytes. The best evidence for <u>in vivo</u> generation of C5a during hemodialysis thus comes from the observation of secondary events that are directly mediated by C5a-C5a receptor interactions such as enhanced expression of CR1 and CR3 receptors on circulating neutrophils (Arnaout et al., 1985) or likely to be mediated by such interactions, e. g. pulmonary hypertension, arterial hypoxia and peripheral leukopenia (Cheung et al., 1986); Craddock et al., 1977). Other consequences of complement activation during hemodialysis including generation of IL-1 (Haeffner-Cavaillon et al., 1989) may be mediated by generated C5a/C5adesArg but also by C3a/C3adesArg which is a less efficient inducer of IL-1 than C5a but is produced in larger amounts during dialysis. Little is known as yet on deleterious effects that could be dependent on the generation of C5b-9 terminal complexes during dialysis with complement-activating membranes.

GENERATION OF INTERLEUKIN-1 (IL-1) DURING HEMODIALYSIS

Fever, generalized malaise, headache and symptomatic hypotension are often observed in hemodialyzed patients (Henderson, 1980; Robinson and Rosen, 1971; Henderson et al., 1983). These symptoms also occurs in patients suffering from infection or inflammatory diseases with ongoing acute phase responses (Dinarello, 1984). Most of the reactions characterizing the acute-phase response are mediated by at least three different cytokines: IL-1, IL-6 and TNF α. Two distinct IL-1 gene products have been cloned, IL-1 α and IL-1 β. Recombinant human IL-1 has been used to confirm the multiple biological properties of the cytokine in vivo including fever (Dinarello and Wolff, 1982), decreased plasma levels of zinc and iron, increased synthesis of acute phase protein in the liver (Ramadozi et al., 1985) stimulation of PGI_2 and platelet activating factor production (Table I).

Many similar changes occur following hemodialysis that were suggested to be dependent on the production of IL-1 (Henderson et al., 1983). IL-1 is produced by human monocytes upon stimulation by a number of substances (Durum et al., 1985), the most relevant to extracorporeal circulation beeing human C5a (C5adesArg), human C3a (C3adesArg) (Haeffner-Cavaillon et al., 1988) and endotoxin or fragments derived therefrom (Haeffner-Cavaillon et al., 1984). IL-1 is not preformed in monocytes and de novo synthesis of RNA and protein occur upon stimulation of the cells. Specific IL-1 mRNA is detected 2h after maximal stimulation of monocytes with LPS. Unlike most secretory proteins both IL-1 α and IL-1 β accumulate intracellularly. The kinetics of IL-1

TABLE 1. FUNCTIONS OF IL-1, IL-6 AND TNF IN THE ACUTE-PHASE REACTION

IN VIVO	IL-1	IL-6	TNF α
Fever, slow-wave sleep, anorexia	++	+	++
Muscle protein and fat degradation	+		++
Acute-phase - protein synthesis	+	++	+
Reduction in blood Zn^{2+} Fe^{2+}	+		+
ACTH release	+		
Hypotension	+		++
Capillary leakage	+		++
Endothelial cell activation	+	+	++

22

TABLE 2.   IN VIVO PRODUCTION OF CELL-ASSOCIATED IL-1 ACTIVITY
           IN MONOCYTES FROM PATIENTS UNDERGOING HEMODIALYSIS
           WITH CUPROPHANE, AN69 AND POLYSULFONE MEMBRANES

| | Monocyte-associated IL-1 U/ml | |
	Start of dialysis (To)	end of dialysis (t=5h)
Cuprophane	12.5 ± 3.0	42.2 ± 5.5
AN69	32.9 ± 5.6	59.2 ± 7.0
Polysulfone	38.0 ± 5.6	36.5 ± 6.7

secretion are unique in comparison with TNF and IL-6: only
50 % of IL-1 β is released following 10hr of culture whereas
no processed IL-1 α is released by the cells (Hazuda et al.,
1988). Stimulation of monocytes with low amounts of LPS
(0.1-1 μg) results in an intracellular accumulation of IL-1
activity; triggering of the cells by C3a (C3adesArg) at
equivalent concentrations to these found in the plasma of
patients undergoing hemodialysis with cellulosic membranes
results in an accumulation of intracellular IL-1 by 6h of
culture in vitro with a maximum at 12h of culture. The
release of IL-1 requires 12-18h of culture. These data suggested that the detection of released IL-1 in plasma during
hemodialysis would virtually be impossible and that a more
suitable assay would be the detection of enhanced intracellular IL-1 activity on freshly isolated monocytes. In order
to evaluate IL-1 activity produced in vivo, the monocyte
content in cytokine should be assessed immediately after the
purification procedure rather than following culture since
monocytes can be activated by the adhesion to plastic. Using
this procedure we have shown that after 5h of hemodialysis
with Cuprophane devices, monocytes from patients produce
biologically active intracellular IL-1 (Table II) (Haeffner-
Cavaillon et al., 1989). Both IL-1 α and IL-1 β antigens
were detected in circulating monocytes during dialysis. In
contrast, little or no intradialytic increase in IL-1
production occured in patients undergoing hemodialysis with
high permeability polyacrylonitrile membranes (Table II).
Results represent the mean ± SEM of cell-associated IL-1
activities measured in uncultured monocytes from 21 patients
dialyzed with Cuprophane membranes, 22 patients dialyzed
with AN69 devices and 16 patients with polysulfone membranes. The mean found in monocytes from 34 normal individuals
was 2.85 ± 0.85 and in monocytes from 10 non-dialyzed patients with chronic renal failure 0.95 ± 0.85 U/ml.

However, in most of the patients chronically dialyzed
with polyacrylonitrile membranes, high levels of monocyte
associated IL-1 were found in predialysis samples. It is
unlikely that the chemical nature of the membrane could be
directly involved in the generation of IL-1 since monocytes
incubated up to 5h with AN69 and polysulfone membranes in
the absence of serum did not produce intracellular IL-1. One
explanation for the high levels of intracellular IL-1
observed in patient dialyzed with high permeability membranes could be transmembrane passage of rough LPS through dialysis membranes. Although dialysis membranes are considered

to be impermeable for LPS, fever during and after hemodialysis has been associated with bacterial contamination in the dialysate (Petersen et al., 1978). Monocytes in fresh human blood circulating through the blood side of a closed-loop dialysis circuit are stimulated to produce IL-1 when endotoxin is present on the dialysate side (Bingel et al., 1986). The assumption that LPS do not cross the membrane is based on the fact that the limulus amebocyte lipage (LAL) test failed to demonstrate a positive reaction (Port et al., 1985). We have however demonstrated that there is a dissociation between the IL-1 inducing capacities and LAL responsiveness of LPS from different origine (Laude, manuscript in preparation, 1989a) and shown that purified radiolabelled LPS cross dialysis membranes and penetrate into the blood compartment in the first minutes of a sham dialysis with AN69 and polysulfone devices. Part of the LPS is beeing trapped in the membrane. Whether trapped LPS is accessible to blood cells and may stimulate IL-1 production is unknown at the present time.

The transient production of complement in patients dialyzed with Cuprophane devices may provide a mechanism for initiating the transient stimulation of IL-1 production. The demonstration of transient perdialytic increase in IL-1 production is another example of the adverse effects that may occur during hemodialysis with complement-bio-incompatible membranes.

The chronic stimulation of IL-1 production in patients hemodialyzed on high permeability membranes may depend on the passage of LPS or on other unidentified factors. The biocompatibility of such membrane for the complement system may thus be counter-balanced by chronic stimulation of IL-1 production. The pathogenic role of IL-1 that may be formed and released transiently or chronically in patients undergoing hemodialysis remains to be proved.

REFERENCES

1. Arnaout, M.A., Hakim, R.M., Todd III, R.F., Dana, N., Colton, H.R.: Increased expression of an adhesion-promoting surface glycoprotein in the granulocytopenia of hemodialysis. New Engl. J. Med. 312:457 (1985).
2. Bhakdi, S., Fassbender, W., Hugo, F., Berstecher, C., Malasit, P., Carreno, M.P., Kazatchkine, M.D.: Relative inefficiency of terminal complement activation. J. Immunol. 144:3117 (1988).
3. Bingel, M., Lonnemann, G. Shaldon, S., Koch, K.M., Dinarello, C.A.: Human IL-1 production during hemodialysis. Nephron 43:161 (1986).
4. Carreno, M.P., Labarre, D., Jozefowicz, M., Kazatchkine, M.D.: The ability of Sephadex to activate human complement is suppressed in specifically substituted functional Sephadex derivatives. Mol. Immunol. 25:165 (1988).
5. Carreno, M.P., Maillet, F., Labarre, D., Jozefowicz, M., Kazatchkine, M.D.: Specific antibodies enhance Sephadex-induced activation of the alternative complement pathway in human serum. Biomaterials 9:514 (1988).

6. Carreno, M.P., Labarre, D. Jozefowicz, M., Kazatchkine, M.D.: Regulation of the human alternative complement pathway: formation of a ternary complex between Factor H, surface-bound C3b and chemical groups on non-activation surfaces. Submitted.

7. Chenoweth, D.E., Cheung, A.K., Ward, D.M., Henderson, L.W.: Anaphylatoxin formation during hemodialysis: effects of different dialyzer membranes. _Kidney_ _Int._ 24:764 (1983).

8. Chenoweth, D.E., Cheung, A.K., Ward., D.M., Henderson, L.W.: Anaphylotoxin formation during hemodialysis: comparison of new and re-used dialyzers. _Kidney_ _Int._ 24:770 (1983).

9. Chenoweth, D.E.: Complement activation during hemodialysis: clinical observations, proposed mechanisms and theoretical implications. _Artif._ _Organs._ 8:281 (1984).

10. Cheung, A.K., Lewinter, M., Chenoweth, D.E., Lew, Y.W., Henderson, L.W.: Cardiopulmonary effects of cuprophan-activated plasma in the Swine: role of complement products. _Kidney_ _Int._ 29:799 (1986).

11. Cheung, A.K., Parker, C.J., Janatova, J.: Analysis of the complement C3 fragments associated with hemodialysis membranes. _Kidney_ _Int._ 35:576 (1989).

12. Craddock, P.R., Fehr, J., Birgham, K.L., Kronenberg, R.S., Jacob, H.S.: Complement and leukocyte-mediated pulmonary dysfunction in hemodialysis. _New_ _Engl._ _J._ _Med._ 296:769 (1977).

13. Dinarello, C.A., Wolff, S.M.: Molecular basis of fever in humans. _Am._ _J._ _Med._ 72:799 (1982).

14. Dinarello, C.A.: Interleukin-1 and the pathogenesis of the acute phase response. _New_ _Engl._ _J._ _Med._ 311:1413 (1984).

15. Durum, S.K., Schmidt, J.A., Oppenheim, J.J.: Interleukin-1: an immunological perspective. _Ann._ _Rev._ _Immunol._ 3:263 (1985).

16. Haeffner-Cavaillon, N., Cavaillon, J.M., Moreau, M., Szabo, L.: Interleukin-1 secretion by human monocytes stimulated by the isolated polysaccharide region of the Bordetella pertusis endotoxin. _Mol._ _Immunol._ 21:389 (1984).

17. Haeffner-Cavaillon, N., Cavaillon, J.M., Cianconi, C., Bacle, F., Delons, S., Kazatchkine, M.D.: C3a (C3ades-Arg) induces production and release of interleukin-1 by cultured monocytes. _J._ _Immunol._ 139:794 (1987).

18. Haeffner-Cavaillon, N., Cavaillon, J.M., Cianconi, C., Bacle, F., Delons, S., Kazatchkine, M.D.: _In vivo_ induction of interleukin-1 production during hemodialysis. _Kidney_ _Int._ 1989 in press.

19. Hakim, R.M., Lowrie, E.G.: Effect of dialyzer reuse on leukopenia, hypoxemia and total hemolytic complement system. _Trans._ _Am._ _Soc._ _Artif._ _Organs_ 26:159 (1980).

20. Hakim, R.M., Breillat, J., Lazarus, J.M., Port, F.K.: Complement activation and hypersensitivity reactions to dialysis membranes. _New_ _Engl._ _J._ _Med._ 311:878 (1984).

21. Hazuda, D.J., La, J.C., Yound, P.R.: The kinetics of interleukin-1 secretion form activated monocytes. _J._ _Biol._ _Chem._ 263:473 (1988).

22. Henderson, L.W.: Symptomatic hypotension during hemodialysis. _Kidney_ _Int._ 17:571 (1980).

23. Henderson, L.W., Koch, K.M., Dinarello, C.A., Shaldon,

S.: Hemodialysis hypotension the hypothesis. <u>Blood</u> <u>Purif.</u> 1:3 (1983).

24. Kazatchkine, M.D., Nydegger, U.E.: The human alternative complement pathway: biology and immunopathology of activation and regulation. <u>Prog.</u> <u>Allergy</u> 30:193 (1982).

25. Moore, F.D., Fearon, D.T., Austen, K.F.: IgG on mouse erythrocytes arguments activation of the human alternative complement pathway by enhancing deposition of C3b. <u>J. Immunol.</u> 126:1805 (1981).

26. Pangburn, M.K.: Mechanisms of recognition of alternative pathway activators: analysis using C3b-bound low-molecular weight polysaccharides of defined structure. Complement (abstract) 4:208 (1987).

27. Petersen, M.J., Boyer, K.M., Carson, L.A., Favero, M.S.: Pyrogenic reactions from inadequate desinfection of a dialysis fluid distribution system. <u>Dialysis</u> <u>Transplant.</u> 7:52 (1978).

28. Port, F.K., Berkick, J.J.: Pyrogen and endotoxin reactions during hemodialysis. <u>Contrib. Nephrol.</u> 36:100 (1983).

29. Ramadoni, G., Sije, J.D., Dinarello, C.A.: Pretranslational modulation of acute phase hepatic synthesis by murine recombinant IL-1 and purified human IL-1. <u>J. Exp. Med.</u> 162:930 (1985).

30. Robinson, P.J.A., Rosen, S.M.: Pyrexial reactions during hemodialysis. <u>Br. Med. J.</u> 1:528 (1971).

31. Schenkein, H.A., Ruddy, S.: The role of immunoglobulins in alternative pathway activation by Zymosan. 1. Human IgG with specificity for Zymosan enhances alternative pathway activation by Zymosan. <u>J. Immunol.</u> 126:7 (1981).

32. Smeby, L.C., Jorstad, S.T., Balstad, T., Wideroe, T.E.: Dialyzer generation and plasma clearance of activated complement during hemodialysis. <u>In:</u> Immune and Metabolic Aspects of Therapeutic Blood Purification systems. Smeby, L.C., Jorstad, S.T. and Wideroe, T.E. (eds.) Karger, Basel p. 76 (1986).

33. Weiss, L., Carreno, M.P., Maillet, F.: Antibody dependency of alternative pathway activation during hemodialysis with cuprophane membrane. Complement (abstract) 5:199.

NEUTROPHIL ACTIVATION DURING HEMODIALYSIS

Marianne Haag-Weber, Peter Schollmeyer,
Walter H. Hörl

Department of Medicine, Division of Nephrology
University of Freiburg, 7800 Freiburg, FRG

INTRODUCTION

Dialyzing membranes are often used in clinical circumstances and are an important factor in the consideration of biocompatibility with non-biological medical paraphernalia. Depending on the unique physical characteristics of the various filters employed, there are some significant side effects regard to cellular activation.

CHEMOTACTIC AND PHAGOCYTOTIC RESPONSIVENESS OF PMN

The chemotactic response of dialyzed polymorphonuclear neutrophils (PMNs) at maximum neutropenia was normal when cuprophan, cellulose acetate, and cellulose hydrate filters were used, whereas their random locomotion was decreased (1). However, the chemotactic response towards agonists was decreased after a single passage through a cuprophan filter (2). Similarly, chemotactic response toward formyl-methionyl-leucyl-phenylalanine (FMLP) was decreased when the cells has been exposed to cellulose membrane (3).

Phagocytotic responsiveness of PMN increased after exposure to cuprophan filter although exposure to polyacrylonitrile and polysulfone hemodialyzers did not affect phagocytotic activity (4). Furthermore, PMN **activation of** glycogenolysis was **increased after** passage through polymethylmethacrylate dialyzer filter that was indicated by an increase of phosphorylase $\underline{a}$ activity (5) as shown in figure 1; in addition, increases in the activities of glycolytic enzymes at the end of hemodialysis treatment have been reported by Metcoff et al. (6). Vanholder et al. (4) observed a dramatic fall in phagocytotic activity after 15 minutes of hemodialysis with cuprophan membranes. Reused cuprophan caused a minor decrease in phagocytotic activity, whereas hemodialysis with polyacrylonitrile and polysulfone produced no significant change in their population. There was a marked increase in the $^{14}CO_2$ production from labeled glucose after 15 minutes of cuprophan hemodialysis but not with the polyacrylonitrile or polysulfone hemodialyzers (7).

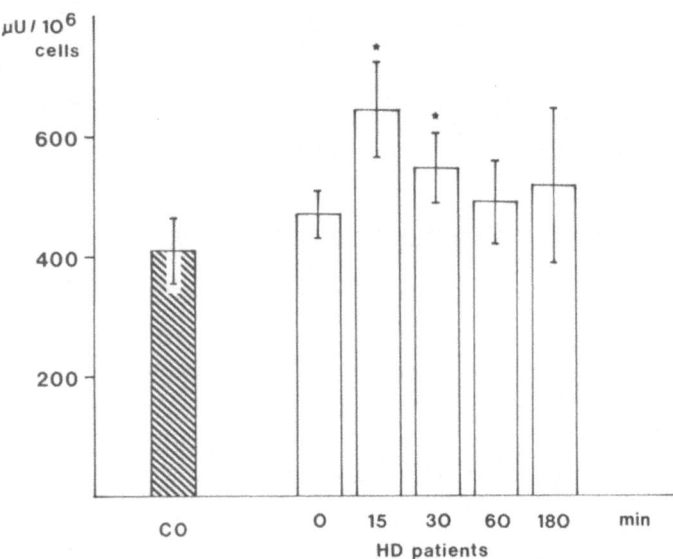

Figure 1. Phosphorylase $\underline{a}$ activity in PMNs of healthy controls and of hemodialysis patients during hemodialysis
*$p < 0.05$ before HD vs during and after HD.

DEGRANULATION

Hemodialysis with cuprophan filter membranes induced C3a and C5a formation, leucopenia, and the gradual release of lactoferrin by PMNs (8). Ivanovich et al. (9) reported an increase of lactoferrin levels during hemodialysis with cuprophan and, to a lesser extent, with cellulose acetate. Hällgren et al. (10) found increased levels of lactoferrin and eosinophilic cationic protein during hemodialysis with cuprophan membranes. However, there was an appreciable binding of lactoferrin and lysozyme to the membrane. Predialysis lysozyme levels were 3 to 4 times higher than in uremic patients (11). Patients dialyzed with cellulose hydrate, cuprophan, or ethylene vinyl alcohol copolymer dialyzers had no significant change in their plasma lysozyme concentration. There was, however, a significant decrease in the plasma lysozyme concentration immediately after hemodialysis when polyacrylonitrile or polymethylmethacrylate membranes were used (11); although others found that lysozyme levels in the afferent blood did not rise (10).

We observed a progressive elevation of plasma elastase in complex with alpha$_1$-proteinase inhibitor (E-alpha$_1$PI) during hemodialysis therapy using dialyzers made of cuprophan (12). Plasma E-alpha$_1$PI levels were higher in diabetic compared with nondiabetic dialysis patients (13). When we studied the effect of different dialyzer membranes on the release of granulocyte elastase, marked differences were observed (11). Similar results were obtained by Knudsen et al. (14). The modified cellulosic membrane (Hemophan) caused lower release of granulocyte elastase and less leukopenia than the regenerated cellulose (Cuprophan) (15). If we compare the results with

28

different membrane materials there is no relationship between initial leukopenia and increased E-alpha$_1$PI levels. Bonal et al. (16) also found no correlation between increased elastase levels and decrease of total leukocyte count.

Granulocyte myeloperoxidase, lactoferrin, collagenase and elastase were released simultaneously following phagocytosis. The release was rapid during the first 10 minutes of phagocytosis, but after 20 minutes the amount of enzyme released increased only slightly. About 25 to 30 % of the granula content of the neutral proteases collagenase and elastase were released to the exterior of the cells, as were similar amounts of myeloperoxidase and lactoferrin (17). On the other hand, plasma levels of the main granulocyte components underwent progressive elevation during hemodialysis (11-15). Furthermore, different amounts of lactoferrin and elastase are released depending on the membrane material of the dialyzer used (18). Specific granules degranulate before azurophilic granules in the presence of immune complexes. In addition, their contents for the greater part leave the PMNs and enter the extracellular fluid. The azurophilc granules degranulate more slowly and their contents, for the greater part, degranulate into phagolysosomes (19).

Studies of Schmidt (20) demonstrated that there is not only differential release of enzymes from azurophilic and specific granules of PMNs, but there also seems to be differential release of the neutral granulocyte proteases elastase and chymotrypsin (cathepsin G), both of which are localized in the primary granules. Elevated plasma myeloperoxidase levels in the presence of each dialyzer demonstrate that none of the membrane are truly biocompatible.

The mechanisms of degranulation of polymorphonuclear leukocytes during hemodialysis are unclear. Significant complement activation and anaphylatoxin formation were observed in patients dialyzed with cuprophan hollow-fiber membranes, whereas polymethylmethacrylate (PMMA) and polyacrylonitrile (PAN) membranes promoted only very little complement activation (9,21-26). Quite possible that active components of C3 and C5 acting as anaphylatoxins are responsible for the granulocyte activation during hemodialysis. However recent studies from our laboratory challenge the concept that neutrophil activation during hemodialysis occurs solely via the activation of the complement pathway. For example, patients dialyzed with cuprophan dialyzers show significant anaphylatoxin formation but only 50 % display **remarkable elevation** of plasma E-alpha$_1$PI levels (27). Thirty chronically uremic patients undergoing regular hemodialysis with dialyzers made of cuprophan were selected in order to compare anaphylatoxin formation and granulocyte lactoferrin release. We could subdivide these patients into four groups. Group I displayed high C3a and low lactoferrin values, group II low C3a and low lactoferrin, group III low C3a and high lactoferrin and group IV high C3a and high lactoferrin. Very little complement activation occurs in patients dialyzed with PMMA but increased plasma levels of main granulocyte components up to 600 % were observed (28). Membranes like PAN are also free of complement-activating potential. However, elevated plasma lactoferrin values indicate degranulation of specific granules under these conditions

(19). Plasma E-alpha$_1$PI levels were significantly higher in patients dialyzed with the polycarbonate compared with the cuprophan membrane. On the other hand, plasma C3a levels were higher in patients dialyzed with the cuprophan dialyzer (29). Recent publications of Schaefer et al. (30) show that release of granulocyte components is strictly dependent on the geometry and the surface of the dialyzer. Plasma levels of E-alpha$_1$PI and lactoferrin were significantly increased during dialysis with flat sheet dialyzers as compared to hollow fiber devices. With respect to surface area, larger dialyzers tend to cause more release of granulocyte constituents as compared to dialyzers with smaller surface areas, irrespective of the configuration of the dialyzer used. Activation of the complement system, however, did not differ with both types of configurations. The same held true for the initial leukopenia (30). Tetta et al. (31) studied the electric properties of membranes and showed that only cationic, but not anionic or neutral PMMA membranes activate plasma-free human PMNs even in the absence of complement. Chenoweth et al. (22) demonstrated that the intensity of complement activation during hemodialysis is determined by the type of dialysis membrane and whether it is new or reused. Reused cuprophan dialyzers displayed very little complement activation (22). Plasma levels of granulocyte lactoferrin and myeloperoxidase, however, remained unchanged even after 10th reuse, whereas 50 % reduction of plasma E-alpha$_1$PI levels were observed (Hörl et al., submitted).

In a study of our laboratory (32) we could demonstrate that the calcium channel blockers nifedipine, diltiazem, verapamil continuously infused during hemodialysis significantly reduced the release of lactoferrin and elastase during hemodialyzers made of PMMA and PAN. The calcium channel blockers had no effect on degranulation of PMNs and anaphylatoxin formation using dialyzers made of cuprophan. Our data indicate that calcium channel blockers inhibit granulocyte activation occuring in dialyzers with very little anaphylatoxin formation. These drugs, however, are ineffective in patients dialyzed with cuprophan where complement activation takes place. Therefore, granulocyte activation during hemodialysis in the absence of complement activation seems to be mediated by calcium ions. Calcium channel blockers reduced degranulation of PMNs also during cardiopulmonary bypass (33) and also in in-vitro experiments (34). A recent study of Betz et al. (35) demonstrates that cuprammonium membranes stimulate interleukin-1 release and arachidonic acid metabolism in monocytes also in the absence of complement.

OXIDATIVE AND CARBOHYDRATE METABOLISM

Different changes in oxidative and carbohydrate metabolism have been observed in PMNs when exposed to a cuprophan filter but not with PAN filter membrane (36). There was a reduced PMN activity of both chemiluminescence (CL) and H_2O_2 as a consequence of hemodialysis when a cuprophan dialyzer was employed; however, the diminished activity was no longer detectable after the filter had been hemophan modified (37). Markert et al. (38) found an increase of phorbol mystrate acetate (PMA)-stimulated lucigenin-amplified CL of PMNs isolated 5 and 60 minutes during hemodialysis with cuprophan, cellulose acetate and PAN during the first and/or second use as compared to the control cells. Luminol increased CL during the initial use of three filters:cuprophan, polycarbonate and polysulfone.

Although numerous studies have affirmed changes of PMN metabolism and function in uremia, most of the evidence has come from data obtained before and during hemodialysis. However, information comparing PMN function after hemodialysis treatment with that prior to treatment are lacking. Studies on glucose metabolism have revealed that glucose intolerance and impaired utilization of glucose are improved significantly after uremic patients have undergone hemodialysis treatment. This suggests that a circulating plasma factor is responsible for inducing insulin resistance (39,40,41). A variety of normal tissues obtained from animals have inhibited basal uptake of glucose following incubation with whole or partially purified sera obtained from uremic patients (42,43,44). The insulin stimulation of glucose uptake and metabolism of rat adipocytes also was reduced following preincubation with serum from uremic patients (45). This irregularity occurs without affecting either insulin binding or the antilipolytic action of insulin (40).

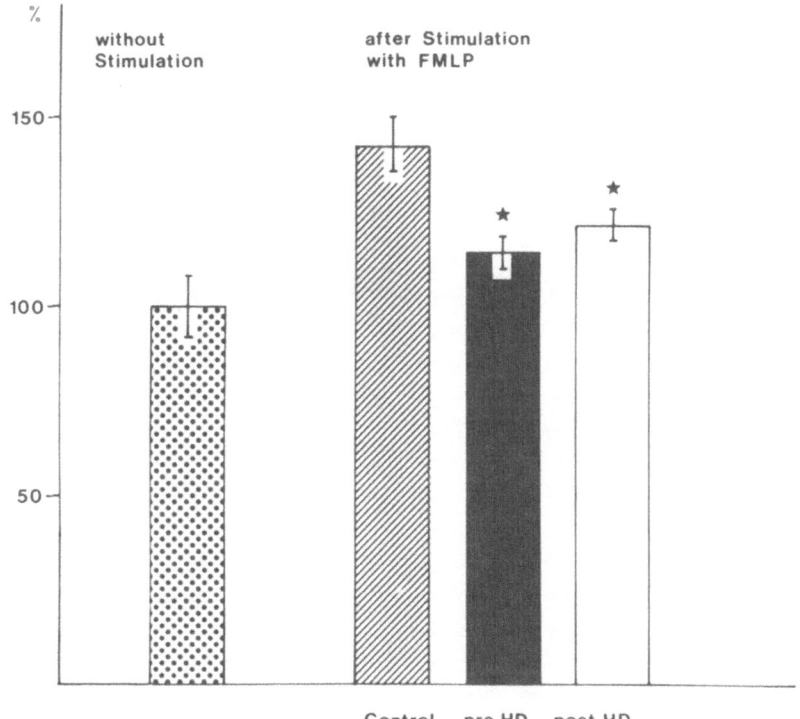

Figure 2. Hexose uptake of PMNs with and without stimulation with FMLP of healthy controls, HD-patients before and after hemodialysis
*p < 0.05 control vs HD-patients

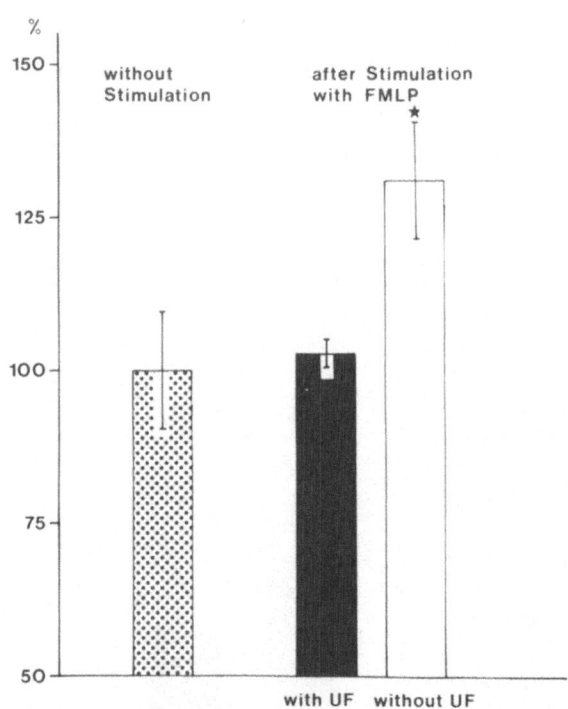

Figure 3. Hexose uptake of PMNs of healthy controls after
stimulation with FMLP with and without ultrafiltrate
of hemodialysis patients
*p< 0.05 without ultrafiltrate vs with ultrafiltrate

Cellular activation of PMN by microbial antigens and certain toxins are achieved by the stimulation of phosphoinositol (PI) turnover and activation of protein kinase C. For example, the stimulus-response coupling in PMN is induced by a chemotactic peptide. Concanavalin A, immune complexes, and PMA showed an increase of calcium uptake preceeding onset of degranulation and of O_2-generation (46). The stimulation of hexose transport by PMNs is associated with the activation of protein kinase C (47). Furthermore, pertussis toxin that is known to involve the activation of G proteins effectively stimulates PI turnover with regard to increased formation of IP_3 and an increased elevation of $(Ca^{2+})i$ (48).

We have observed recently that PMNs from uremic patients have diminished responsiveness to FMLP-induced hexose uptake, enzyme release, and chemotaxis (49). As shown in figure 2 this lack of responsiveness is improved after the patients have undergone hemodialysis. Moreover, when normal PMN are exposed to various concentrations of ultrafiltrates from uremic patients, there was an increased loss of responsiveness of these cells with regard to hexose uptake (figure 3) and enzyme release. In addition, washing the PMN with buffered saline restored their function to normal which suggests that a plasma-derived constituent is responsible for these effects. There is further evidence for the existence of such a putative entity from initial experiments that have employed one species with a 8-30 kDa MW that was purified by column chromatography (Sephadex G-100) from the ultrafiltate of uremic patients. The factor appears to be heat stable which suggests that it can be further purified, characterized and its biochemical and immunochemical properties further elucidated.

SUMMARY

Oxidative metabolism of PMNs of uremic patients is enhanced due to unknown serum (plasma) factors which are removed during hemodialysis. Respiratory burst activity is diminished in both PMA-stimulated and unstimulated states compared to healthy controls. Hemodialysis normalizes stimulated and decreases unstimulated hydrogen peroxide production. Several authors found that resting and stimulated chemiluminescence (CL) during hemodialysis correlates with complement activation, whereas other authors describe CL using dialyzer membranes with only mild anaphylatoxin formation. Alterations of PMN carbohydrate metabolism in uremic patients improves during HD with polysulfone. HD with PMMA, however, activates glycogenolysis. These alterations may be responsible for disturbance in phagocytosis. Degranulation during HD also occurs in absence of complement activation. Calcium channel blockers decrease activation of PMNs using dialyzers with only little anaphylatoxin formation.

REFERENCES

1. A. Losito, V. Buoncristiani and C. Cecchini, Abnormal leucocyte locomotion induced by hemodialysis membranes, A clue to dialysis leukopenia. J Clin Lab Immunol 10:87 (1983)
2. B. Wierusz-Wysocka, H. Wysocki, R. Czarnecki, H. Siekierka, B. Kazimierz and K. Wysocki, Influence of hemodialysis on plasma chemotactic responsiveness of polymorphonuclear neutrophils. Artif Organs 7:159 (1983)
3. W. Marker, P.A. Waridel, C. Heierli and J.P, Wauters. Neutrophil functions during hemodialyis. Contrib Nephrol 62:99 (1988)
4. R.C: Vanholder, A. Dhondt and S.M.G. Ringoir, Challenge of phagocyte metabolism by extracorporeal circulation and membrane contact: A biocompatible test. Trans Am Soc Artif Intern Organs 34:214 (1988)
5. M. Haag-Weber, G. Fiedler, P. Schollmeyer and W.H. Hörl, Activation of neutrophil glycogenolysis during hemodialysis. Blood (submitted for publication)
6. J. Metcoff, R. Lindemann, D. Baxter and J. Peterson, Cell metabolism in uremia. Am J Clin Nutr 30:1627 (1978)
7. B. Descamps-Latscha, Phagocyte oxidative metabolism in hemodialysis. Contrib Nephrol 62:132 (1988)
8. D.E. Chenoweth, The properties of human C5a anaphylatoxins: The significance of C5a formation during hemodialysis. Contr Nephrol 59:51 (1987)
9. P. Ivanovich, D.E. Chenoweth, R. Schmidt, H. Klinkmann, L.A. Boxer, H.S. Jacobs and D.E. Hammerschmidt, Symptoms and activation of granulocytes and complement with two dialyzer membranes. Kidney Int 24:758 (1983)
10. R. Hällgren, P. Venge and B. Willström, Hemodialysis -induced increase in serum lactoferrin and serum eosinophil cationic protein as signs of local neutrophil and eosinophil degranulation. Nephron 29: 233 (1981)
11. W.H. Hörl, H.B. Steinhauer and P. Schollmeyer, Plasma levels of granulocyte elastase during hemodialysis: effects of different dialyzer membranes. Kidney Int 28:791 (1985)
12. W.H. Hörl, M. Jochum, A. Heidland and H. Fritz, Release of granulocyte proteinases during hemodialysis. Am J Nephrol 3:213 (1983)
13. W.H. Hörl, R.M. Schaefer, C. Wanner, J. Bahlmann, J. Reitinger, P. Schollmeyer and A. Heidland, Enhanced plasma and intracellular levels of main granulocyte components in diabetics on dialysis. Blood Purif (in press)
14. F. Knudsen, A.H. Nielsen and P.O. Pedersen, Leukopenia and release of granulocyte elastase: interlinked membrane -dependent events during hemodialysis. Blood Purif 2:36 (1984)
15. R.M. Schaefer, W.H. Hörl, K. Kokot and A. Heidland, Enhanced biocompatibility with a new cellulosic membrane: Cuprophan versus Hemophan. Blood Purif 5:262 (1987)

16. J. Bonal, C. Pastor, J Teixido, J Bonet, A. Serra, R. Lauzurica, R. Romero, A. Caralps and A. Corominas, Plasma levels of granulocyte elastase:its role on the assessment of hemodialysis membrane biocompatibility (abstract) Kidney Int 30:129 (1986)

17. K. Ohlsson and I. Ohlsson, Neutral proteases of human granulocytes. III: Interaction between human granulocyte elastase and plasma protease inhibitors. Scand J Clin Lab Invest 34:349 (1974)

18. W.H. Hörl, W. Riegel, H.B. Steinhauer, C. Wanner, F Thaiss, F. Bozkurt, M. Haag and P. Schollmeyer, Granulocyte activation during hemodialysis. Clin Nephrol 26 (Suppl 1):S-30 (1986)

19. J.K. Spitznagel, Intracellular and extracellular degranulation of human polymorphonuclear azurophil and specific granules induced by immune complexes, in: "Neutral Proteases of Human Polymorphonuclear Leukocytes", K. Havemann and A. Janoff, eds., Urban & Schwarzenberg, Baltimore-Munich (1978)

20. W. Schmidt, Differential release of elastase and chymotrypsin from polymorphonuclear leukocytes, in: "Neutral Proteases of Human Polymorphonuclear Leukocytes", K. Havemann and A. Janoff, eds., Urban & Schwarzenberg, Baltimore-Munich (1978)

21. D.E. Chenoweth, A.K. Cheung and L.W. Henderson, Anaphylatoxin formation during hemodialysis: effects of different dialyzer membranes. Kidney Int 24:764 (1983)

22. D.E. Chenoweth, A.K. Cheung, D.M. Ward and L.W. Henderson, Anaphylatoxin formation during hemodialysis: comparison of new and re-used dialyzers. Kidney Int 24:770 (1983)

23. D.E. Chenoweth, Complement activation during hemodialysis: clinical observations, proposed mechanisms, and theoretical implications. Artif Organs 8:281 (1984)

24. A.K. Cheung and L.W. Henderson, Effects of complement activation by hemodialysis membranes. Am J Nephrol 6:81 (1986)

25. R.M. Hakim, D.T. Fearon and J.M. Lazarus, Biocompatibility of dialysis membranes: effect of chronic complement activation. Kidney Int 26:194 (1984)

26. R.M. Hakim, J. Breillatt, J.M. Lazarus and F.K. Port, Complement activation and hypersensitivity reactions to dialysis membranes. N Engl J Med 311:878 (1984)

27. W.H. Hörl and A. Heidland, Evidence for the participation of granulocyte proteinases on intradialytic catabolism. Clin Nephrol 21:314 (1984)

28. W.H. Hörl, W. Riegel, P. Schollmeyer, W. Rautenberg and S. Neumann, Different complement and granulocyte activation in patients dialyzed with PMMA dialyzers. Clin Nephrol 25:304 (1986)

29. W.H. Hörl, W. Riegel and P. Schollmeyer, Plasma levels of main granulocyte components in patients dialyzed with polycarbonate and cuprophan membranes. Nephron 45:272 (1987)

30. R.M. Schaefer, A. Heidland and W.H. Hörl, Effect of dialyzer geometry on granulocyte and complement activation. Am J Nephrol 7:121 (1987)

31. C. Tetta, G. Camussi, G. Segoloni and A. Vercellone, Direct interaction between polymorphonuclear neutrophils (PMN) and dialysis membranes: role of the electrical charges (abstract). Kidney Int 29:609 (1986)

32. M. Haag-Weber, P. Schollmeyer and W.H. Hörl, Granulocyte activation in the absence of complement activation: inhibition by calcium channel blockers. Eur J Clin Invest 18:380 (1988)

33. W. Riegel, G. Spillner, V. Schlosser and W.H. Hörl, Plasma levels of main granulocyte components during cardiopulmonary bypass. J Thorac Cardiovasc Surg 95:1014 (1988)

34. K. Kokot, M Teschner, R.M. Schaefer and A. Heidland, Stimulation and inhibition of elastase release from human neutrophil-dependence on the calcium messenger system. Mineral Electrolyte Metab 13:189 (1987)

35. M. Betz, G.M. Haenisch, E.W. Rauterberg, J. Bommer and E. Ritz, Cuprammonium membranes stimulate interleukin-1 release and arachidonic acid metabolism in monocytes in the absence of complement. Kidney Int 34:67 (1988)

36. A.T. Nguyen, C. Lethias, J. Zingraff, A. Herbelin, C. Naret and B. Descamps-Latscha, Hemodialysis membrane -induced activation of phagocyte oxidative metabolism detected in vivo and in vitro within microamounts of whole blood. Kidney Int 28:158 (1985)

37. G. Kolb, H. Schönemann, W. Fischer, K. Bittner, H. Lange, H. Höffken, V. Damann, K. Joseph and K. Havemann, Hemodialysis with cuprophan membranes lead to alteration of granulocyte oxidative metabolism and leucocyte sequestrion in the lung, in: "Proteases: Potential Role in Health and Disease II", W.H. Hörl and A. Heidland, eds., Plenum, New York, p 2 (1988)

38. M. Markert, C. Heierli, T. Kuwahara, J. Frei and J.P. Wauters, Dialyzed polymorphonuclear neutrophil oxidative metabolism during dialysis: a comparative study with 5 new and reused membranes. Clin Nephrol 29:129 (1988)

39. M.L. McCaleb, M.S. Izzo and D.H. Lockwood, Characterization and partial purification of a factor from uremic human serum that induces insulin resistance. J Clin Invest 75:391 (1985)

40. R.A. DeFronzo, J.D. Tobin, J.W. Rowe and R. Andres, Glucose intolerance in uremia. J. Clin Invest 62:425 (1978)

41. C.L. Hampers, J.S. Soeldner, P.B. Doak and J.P. Merrill, Effect of chronic renal failure and hemodialysis on carbohydrate metabolism. J. Clin Invest 45:1719 (1966)

42. P. Balestri, P. Rindi, M. Biagini and S. Giovanetti, Effects of uraemic serum, urea, creatinine and methylguanidine on glucose metabolism. Clin Sci 42:395 (1972)

43. J.M. Morgan and R.E. Morgan, Study of the effect of uremic metabolites on erythrocyte glycolysis. Metab Clin Exp 13:629 (1964)

44. R. Dzurik, Metabolic alterations caused by uremia. Proc Eur Dial Transplant Assoc 17:577 (1980)

45. M.L. McCaleb, R. Mevorach, R.B. Freeman, M.S. Izzo and D.H. Lockwood, Induction of insulin resistance in normal adipose tissue by uremic serum. Kidney Int 25:416 (1984)

46. H.M. Korchak, L.E. Rutherford and G. Weissmann, Stimulus response coupling in the human neutrophils. I. Kinetic analysis of changes in calcium permeability. J Biol Chem 259:4070 (1984)

47. Ch. McCall, J. Schmitt, S. Cousart, J. O'Flaherty, D. Bass and R. Wykle, Stimulation of hexose transport by human polymorphonuclear leucocytes: a possible role of protein kinase C. Biochem Biophys Res Comm 126:450 (1985)

48. K.H. Krause, W. Schlegel, C.B. Wollheim, T. Andersson, F.A. Waldvogel and P.D. Lew, Chemotactic peptide activation of human neutrophils and HL-60 cells. Pertussis toxin reveals correlation between inositol triphophate generation, calcium ion transients, and cellular activation. J. Clin Invest 76:1348 (1985)

49. M. Haag-Weber, M. Hable, P. Schollmeyer and W.H. Hörl, Hemodialysis improves carbohydrate metabolism in polymorphonuclear neutrophils (PMN) (abstract). Kidney Int 35:248 (1989)

BIOCOMPATIBILITY - A SYSTEM APPROACH

Horst Klinkmann and Dieter Falkenhagen

Dept. Internal Medicine, Wilhelm Pieck University
DDR-2500 Rostock, German Democratic Republic

INTRODUCTION

The use of more than 2 billion biomaterial devices per year in therapeutic medicine elucidates the magnitude of one of the biggest problems today's medicine is dealing with. Clinical application of biomaterials has by far exceeded in both quality and quantity our knowledge about the interaction between the biomaterial and the human organism (1).

Since ultimately almost every human in technologically advanced societies will host a biomaterial, the incompatibility of this biomaterial will often be catastrophic for the individual.

Therefore complications ranging from simple indisposition to fatalities must be related to our ignorance about several basic facts of this interaction or our poor understanding or even misinterpretation of the results of theoretical work and basic research.

Out of this general frustration and partially ignorance the quality concept of biomaterials has been developed and termed biocompatibility. However this quality concept did not escape the greatest danger to basic research in our days - the desire for immediate success of its clinical application (2).

It will be the aim of this contribution to present a certainly biased view on this obvious problem of open questions and misinterpretations, based upon the use of the artificial kidney in the treatment of end-stage renal failure. No attempt is made to review the total subject but rather to demonstrate the danger of premature interpretation of isolated results for its clinical relevance in a biological system - the human organism (3).

TERMINOLOGY

   Almost all of the biomaterials used in medicine today
are derived from industrial developments for non-medical
purpose. Since the term "biomaterial" is generally applied
to natural or synthetic material that is used in contact
with living tissue and/or biological fluids, a concept was
required to judge the quality of these materials. Until the
late 70's hemolysis and thrombogenicity caused by the relevant biomaterial remained the prevailing parameters for
judging the quality of that material. For this blood-
material interaction with the protein on the material
surfaces as a dominant feature the term "hemocompatibility"
was introduced, and different in vitro and in vivo methods
for assessments developed (4,5). The almost revolutionary
increase in the utilization of biomaterials in medicine
during the last 15 years has caused a tremendous development
in their characterisation - requirements for these materials
in order to target the most suitable biomaterials for its
intended application. Various attempts were made to eluci-
date in addition to the blood-material interaction also the
material-tissue interaction and the involvement of the
immune-system, including cellular and humoral responses to
the material. These numerous results of different origin
were than put together under the collective and descriptive
title of "Biocompatibility".

   From the time of its introduction the term biocompatibility is characterized as an interfacial problem of high
complexity between a nonbiological surface and a living
system. It comprises the energetics and kinetics of all
physical, chemical and biochemical processes at the interface between the material and the biological system during
and after the time of contact as well as the acute and
chronic reactions of the biological system induced by these
processes (6).

   In 1984 our group reviewed this complex interfacial
problem from a simple clinical point of view, taking mainly
into consideration the short and long term effects of

Table 1 Biocompatibility characteristics

- The energetics and kinetics of all physical, chemical,
   and biochemical processes at the interface between the
   biomaterial and the biological system

- The direct reaction of the biological system induced by
   these processes at the interface

- The sum of changes of physical and chemical properties of
   the material, i. e. surface composition, surface free
   energy, corrosion, biodegradation, ect.

- The sum of changes of the biological system outside the
   interface, triggered or induced by the interaction (toxic
   or immune reactions, cancer, ect.)

Table 2 NO-Definition of biocompatibility

- thrombogenic, toxic, allergic, inflammatory reaction

- destruction of formed elements

- changes in plasma proteins and enzymes

- immunological reaction

- carcinogenic effect

- deterioration of adjacent tissues

---

biomaterials on the human organism. This resulted in the so-called NO-definition, which is now gaining wide acceptance in the medical community (6).

Nevertheless, due to the poorly understood high complexity of the biocompatibility scenario and the unavailability of an internationally accepted definition there was and still is an uncritical mixture of terminology initiating a stream of misleading conclusions. This is today quite obvious in the field of blood-purification devices, where on merely practical grounds hemocompatibility and biocompatibility are used as identical terms not according to science but according to convenience and for reasons of marketing competitions.

The compounds cannot be separated from the material

Since the work of Craddock et al. (7) in 1977, the complement system has been widely investigated and is very often used as a quality marker for biocompatibility of a dialyzer (8,9,10,11).

The clinical interest stems from the discussion that complement-material interaction may cause a production or stimulating of inflammatory mediation and may contribute to pathophysiologic alteration in the exposed patient (12,13).

Detailed descriptions of the complement system and its activation can be found in various reviews (14,15) as well as its reported clinical consequences.

In dialysis the extent of complement activation is generally related to the membrane-material. The classical dialysis membrane, Cuprophan, consisting of regenerated cellulose, has been charged with the highest incidence of complement activation and cellulosic membranes were often regarded as lesser biocompatible than other polymeric membranes (16,17). Based upon basic research we know however that the complement activation is related to the chemical compounds of the membrane-material (polysaccharide)

Table 3 Direct biological activity of
complement activation

---

1.   Releasing of : biological active substances from
                    cell granules
                  : thrombokinase from platelets
                  : lysosomal enzymes from granulocytes
                    and B-lymphocytes

2.   Opsonization of bacteria and viruses

3.   Immune adherence of neutrophiles, monocytes,
     B-lymphocytes, macrophages

4.   Stimulation of antibody production of lymphocytes

5.   Membrane lysis of bacteria, viruses, tumor- und
     endothel cells

---

and to the hydroxyl groups. In an attempt to block these
reactive hydroxyl groups of the cellulose OH^- groups were
replaced with amino groups (Hemophan[R]) (18).

   This results in a significant decrease in complement
activation. A similar result can be achieved by replacing
hydroxyl groups by acetate (cellulose acetate).

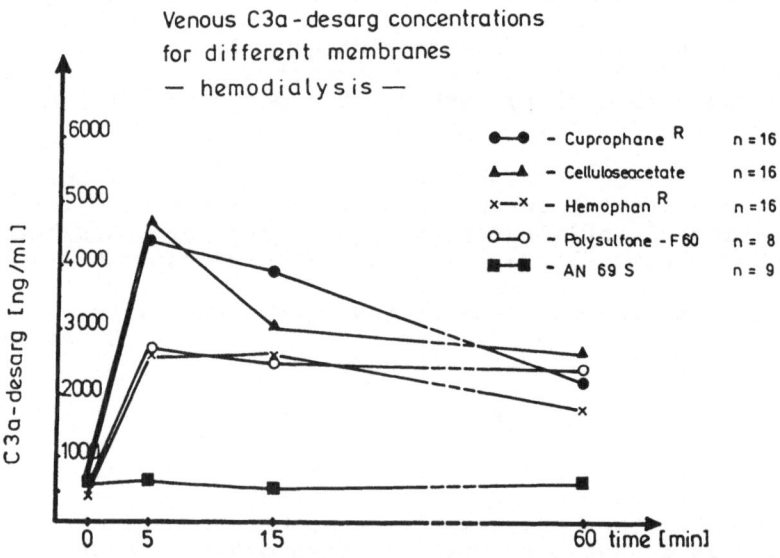

Venous C3a-desarg concentrations
for different membranes
— hemodialysis —

Fig. 1 Comparison of C3a generation during dialysis in
        three different cellulosic membranes and two non-
        cellulosic membranes

Table 4   Standardized white blood cell (WBC) drop in
           relation to surface area in dialysis procedure
           after 10 min (Cuprophan, dog)

Surface area (sqm)	Membrane thickness (um)	WBC (Gpt/l)
0.1	11	7.2±2.1
0.2	11	5.3±2.0
0.4	11	4.6±2.3
0.6	11	4.5±2.2

This documents that a relatively small change in the
compounds can alter the biocompatibility of a basic material
considerably (19).

The material cannot be separated from the device

Clinical observations with different membrane surface
area dialyzers indicated a relationship between WBC-drop,
complement activation and the membrane contact area.

Results obtained by us in experimental studies by using
dialyzers with Cuprophan-membranes of different surface
areas (0.1 to 0.6 m², wall thickness 11 µm) and a newly
developed experimental Cuprophan dialyzer (0.6 m², 5 µm)
demonstrate, that the WBC-drop is proportional to the membrane contact area (20).

An often ignored impact on biocompatibility is that of
the geometric design of the device. Flow geometry and therefore shear stress is different in hollow fibre or flat-sheet
dialyzer. Using the same membrane (Cuprophan[R]) in devices
with different geometric design (G 10 - 3 N hollow fiber,
G 120 M plate dialyzer) a significant difference in platelet
aggregation is apparent, clearly favoring the plate device
(fig. 2).

Both examples demonstrate clearly that biocompatibility
of a material can change significantly depending upon the
device in which the material is used.

The device cannot be separated from the procedure

When measured at the outlet, dialyzers with different
polymeric membranes with larger pore size like polysulfone
or polyacrylonitrile displace a lesser degree of complement
activation (21,22). Not questioning different material properties as a possible reason, the molecular weight of 10,000
dalton of the C3a complement factor indicates the possibility of filtration of complement components in membranes
with larger pore size.

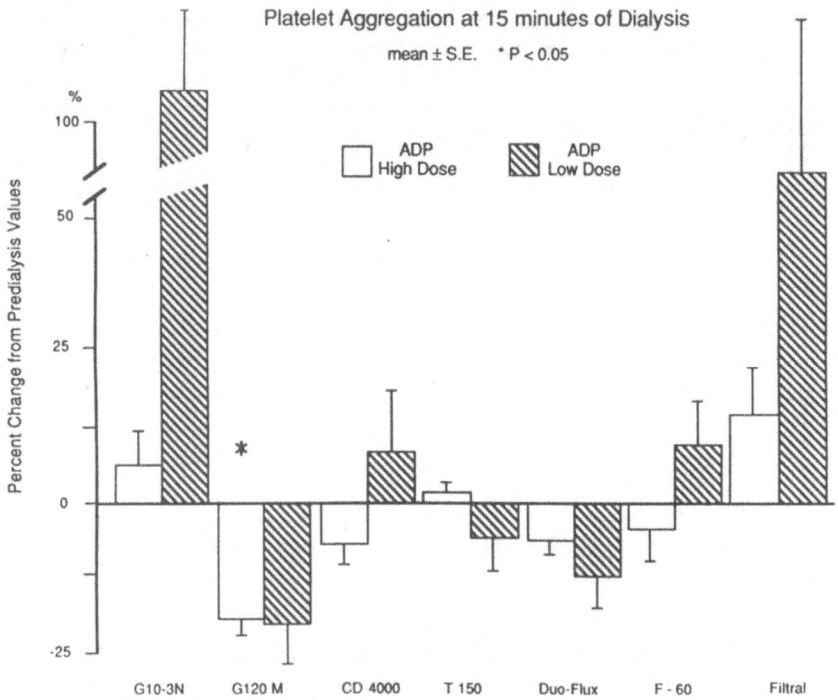

Fig. 2 Differences in platelet aggregation due to different
dialyzer geometry in dialysers with the same
material (G 120-M cuprophan hollow fibre, G 10-3 N
cuprophan plate). All the other devices used for the
comparison are hollow fibre kidneys with different
membranes.

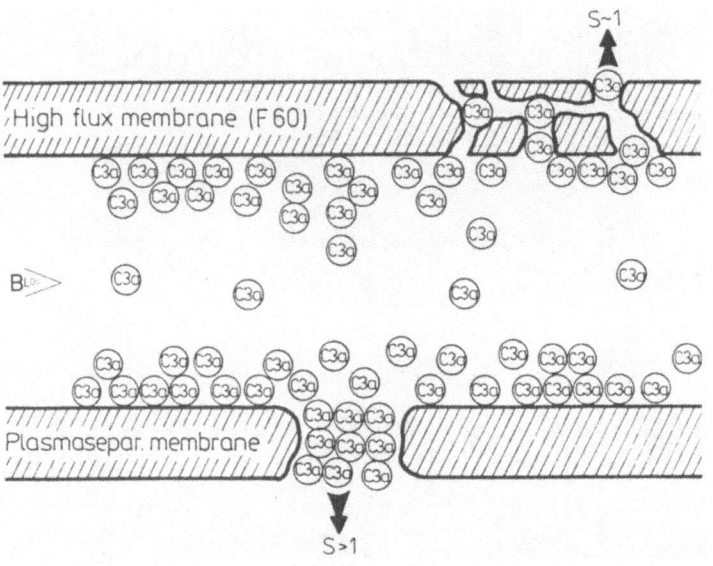

Fig. 3 Schematic diagram to demonstrate complement
filtration through large pore size membranes.

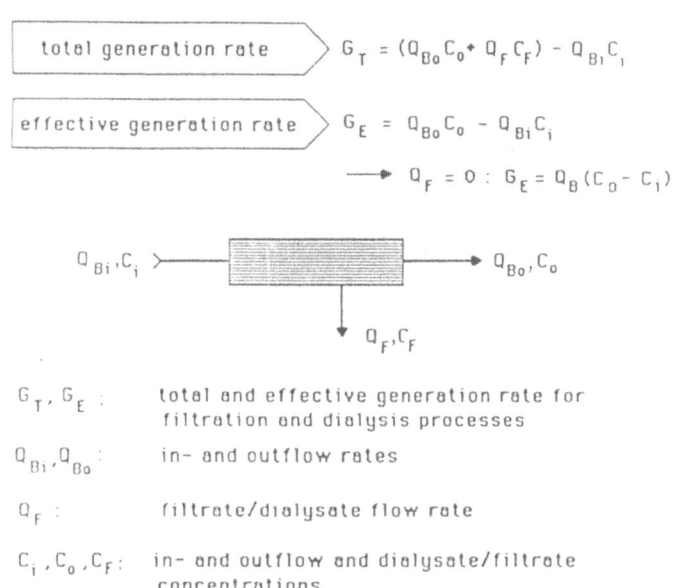

$$G_T = (Q_{Bo}C_o + Q_F C_F) - Q_{Bi}C_i$$

$$G_E = Q_{Bo}C_o - Q_{Bi}C_i$$

$$\longrightarrow Q_F = 0 : G_E = Q_B(C_o - C_i)$$

$G_T, G_E :$ total and effective generation rate for filtration and dialysis processes

$Q_{Bi}, Q_{Bo} :$ in- and outflow rates

$Q_F :$ filtrate/dialysate flow rate

$C_i, C_o, C_F :$ in- and outflow and dialysate/filtrate concentrations

Fig. 4 Total and effective anaphylatoxin generation rate

Based upon our results there is clear evidence, that complement components generated by different membranes, can be abandoned by filtration through the membrane before entering the patient (23).

We therefore suggest to consider for further studies the differences between the total generation rate of a substance, which derives from the device, and the final amount that finally enters the human organism, termed effective generation rate (3).

Our study of one device, equipped with the same membrane (polysulfone) revealed clearly that biocompatibility of the same device varies considerably if the device is used in different modes of application. Used in the dialyzer mode the **larger pore-size of the device is less effective** and therefore the effective generation rate comes closer to the total generation rate. Using the polysulfone membrane as a hemofilter, the larger pore-size becomes more effective. As a result of the filtration there is a large difference between the total and effective generation data.

Thus biocompatibility of a device depends also on the procedure with which the device is operated. Evidence for this is also given by the interleukin-I (IL-1) hypothesis as postulated by Shaldon et al. (24).

IL-1, formerly known as endogenous pyrogen is a monocyte hormone which mediates fever and influences possibly the acute phase response resulting in hepatic synthesis of C-reactive protein, amyloid-A-like substances

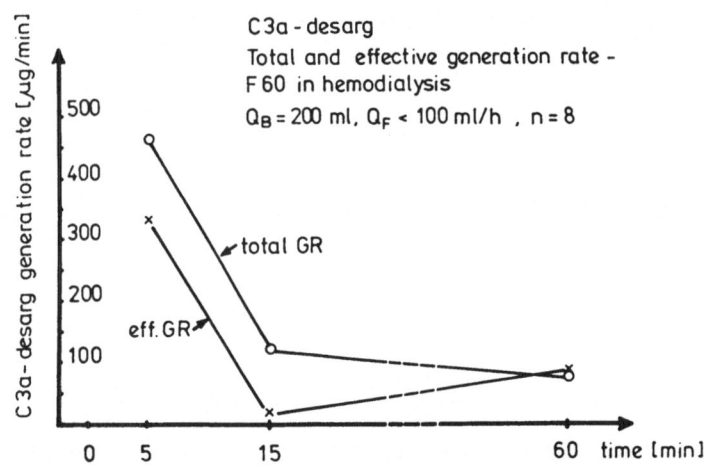

Fig. 5 Total (circle) and effective (crosses) generation
rate of C3a des Arg in the F 60 polysulfone device
used in the dialysis mode.

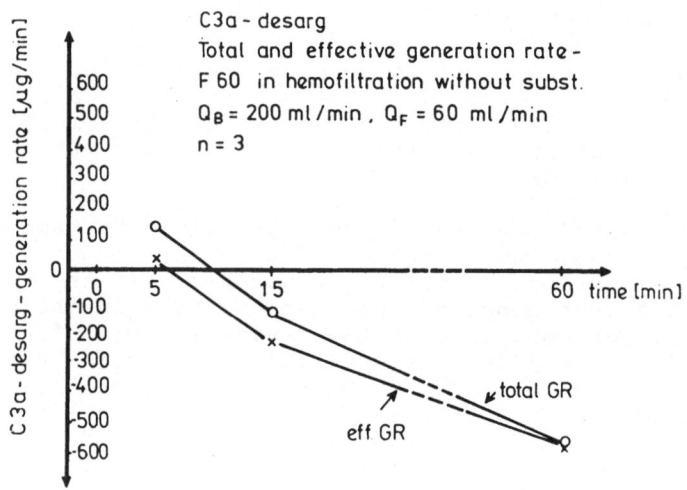

Fig. 6 Total (crosses) and effective (circle) generation
rate of C3a des Arg in the F 60 polysulfone device
in the hemofiltration mode.

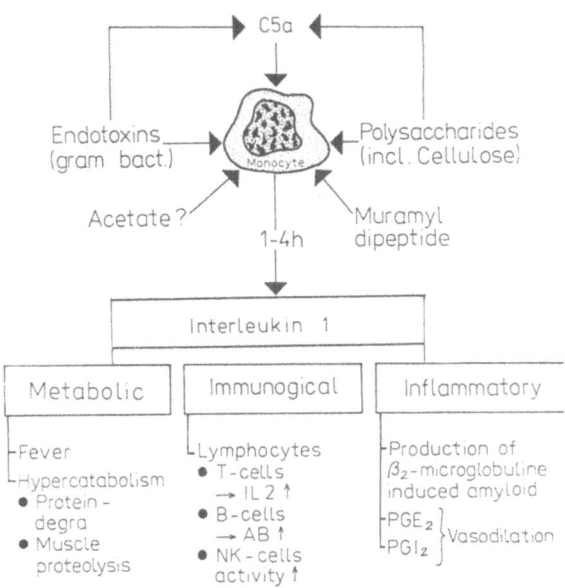

Fig. 7 Biological activity of interleukin-I (IL-I)

and muscle breakdown with hypercatabolism. During dialysis,
monocytes adhere to the membrane in different quantity
according to the type of membrane material used. They are
than exposed to activated complement components and ag-
gregated granulocytes from the blood-side. Additionally
other inducers deriving directly from the dialysate
(endotoxin from gram neg. bacteria, acetate etc.) seemed to
have also an influence. Therefore the total system of the
blood detoxification device has been considered as a
bioreactor, which varies considerably in its activity
according to the specific procedure. For example, the
hemofiltration-mode with the missing dialysate-side and a
pyrogen-free substitution solution seems to cause less IL-I
production than conventional dialysis treatment (25).

Clinically the repeated stimulation of IL-I during
years of treatment could be responsible for acutely induced
vasodilation with hypotension, sleep tendency and even protein catabolism. Long term complications such as osteopenia,
fibrosis and amyloidosis are also related to repeated
stimulation of IL-I (26).

The procedure cannot be separated from the patient

There is convincing evidence, that the individuality of
the specific patient at the time of application of the procedure has an important effect upon the actual and chronic
reaction of the human organism. Since this probably most important factor for the clinical relevance has been almost
neglected in numerous studies on biocompatibility we conducted an international study in different continents with different ethnical groups and different conditions. The complete results of this study, will be published else where.

They support convincingly that geographical, cultural, ethnical and even economical differences may have a much greater influence on the biocompatibility of a treatment procedure as considered earlier and may well explain the big differences in clinical observations with regard to biocompatibility as reported in literature.

The ongoing discussion on the clinical importance of beta$_2$-microglobulin (mol. mass 11,800 daltons) may serve as an example for this statement. Beta$_2$-microglobulin is normally present in plasma and accumulates obviously in blood of uremic patients. Amyloid-like deposits in skin, bone, synovia etc. causing severe clinical complications, have been observed in long term dialysis patients (27). With the detection of beta$_2$-microglobulin in the amyloid fibrils in dialysis-associated amyloidosis (28) in connection with the reported differences in the removal rate by different membranes, beta$_2$-microglobulin seemed to emerge as an important marker of biocompatibility with clinical relevance.

Comparison of available data in literature however demonstrate clearly, that neither the biocompatibility of the membrane-material nor the device or the procedure can be significantly accounted for this clinically important long term complication. It emerges from most of the data, that most likely the patient with his residual renal function, his response to the treatment related induction of monokine production, the disturbances in his iron-metabolism, individual differences in preexisting beta$_2$-microglobulin as well as preexisting pathology in lokalised parts of the organism with local enrichment, local failure of degradation or even local generation, is the determining factor in the beta$_2$-microglobulin story. This subject was recently reviewed in depth by Ritz and Bommer (29) and Flöge et al. (30).

Biostability

Having discussed biocompatibility as a system-approach in the treatment of kidney failure we must recognize, that the meaning of biocompatibility is quite differently understood in the different fields of artificial organ therapy even if the basic biomaterial used is the same. Considering the term biocompatibility as an overall quality marker for a therapeutic system in its complex relation to the patient, the stability of this system becomes very important. Modes of biocompatibility failure include biodegradation as well as material related infections. The perturbation of the host-defence system by a biomaterial and the triggering of local as well as general reactions do influence the biostability of both systems, the patient and the therapeutic device.

One of the features of biostability and consequently biocompatibility will soon be the biomaterial centered infection. A microscopic defect on the material surface favors the interaction between the bacteria and the biomaterial.

Table 5 Main factors determining biostability

Biodegradation

- negative change of mechanical properties

- surface erosion (leaching)

- molecular chain disruption (f. c. hydrolysis)

- chemical imbalances (calcification)

Biomaterial related infection

- microbial colonization of biomaterial

- biomaterial-dependent change in pathogenicity
  of bacteria

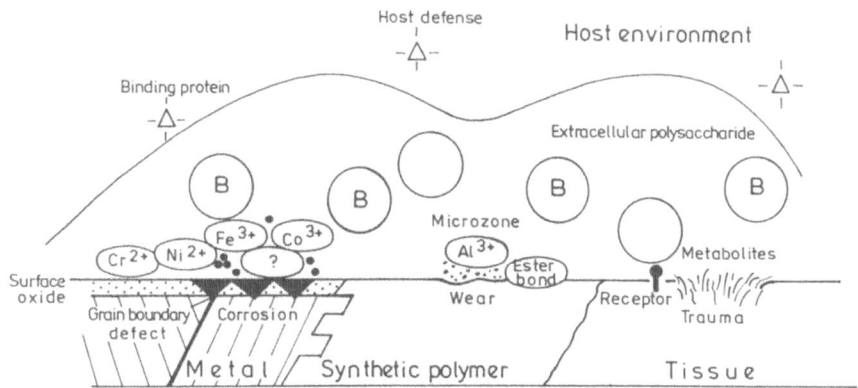

Fig. 8 Interaction between bacteria (B) and biomaterial
        (metal, covered with synthetic polymer).

Fig. 8 demonstrates this situation for a metal base covered with a polymeric surface. Atomic geometry and electronic state as well as unsatisfied bonds of the material are the binding site of the bacterial cell. Polysaccharide polymers, proteinaceus adhesin (fimbria) and other surface and milieu-interieur substances interact and form an aggregate of these different substances in a secondary layer (biofilm) on the surface, which is the basis of biocompatibility of that biomaterial for its interaction with the organism.

Recent studies indicate even a direct influence of the biomaterial upon the pathogenicity of a microorganism. There is even a certain specifity among the bacteria in regard to their preferred material. When the biomaterial is a polymer, Staphylococcus epidermis is frequently involved, whereas Staphylococcus aureus is often the pathogen in biometals (31).

An understanding of these mechanisms is of growing importance to the overall concept of biocompatibility and might soon become its key issue.

Conclusion

The quality concept of biocompatibility has been developed out of the general need to classify biomaterials for medical use but also under partially ignorance of basic research. This quality concept did not escape the greatest danger of todays science - the desire for immediate success of its application. In the mid-70th biocompatibility was already accepted as the main factor in the design of artificial organs and internationally agreed methodology and definition was only a short time away. With todays wealth of information available, this agreement seems to be much further away.

Increased knowledge coupled with sometimes very diverse views, misinterpretation and an uncritical mixture of data and terminology initiated premature and misleading conclusions for clinical relevance. Our human organism is an ancient and highly adaptive biological system. Biocompatibility of an artificial organ, which is designed to fit into this biological system, can only become a true quality concept, if it is applied as a system approach.

REFERENCES

1. Klinkmann, H.: The role of biomaterials in the application of artificial organs. In: Paul, J.P., Gaylor, J.D.S., Courtney, J.M., Gilchrist, T. (eds.), Biomaterial in Artificial Organs, p. 1, Macmillan, London (1984).
2. Szycher, M.: Thrombosis, hemostasis, and thrombolysis at prosthetic interfaces. In: Szycher, M. (ed.), Biocompatible Polymers, Metals, and Composites, p. 1, Technomic Publ. Co., Lancaster, Pennsylvania (1983).
3. Klinkmann, H., Falkenhagen, D., Courtney, J.M.: Clinical relevance of biocompatibility. "The material cannot

be divorced from the device". In: Nefrologia, Vol.VII. Suplemento 3: 13 (1987).

4. Bjornson, J.: Thrombus formation in the artificial kidney. Scand. J. Urol. Nephrol. 12:251 (1978).
5. Wilson, R.D., Lelah, M.D., Cooper, S.L.: Blood-material interactions: Assessment of in-vitro and in-vivo test methods. In: Williams, D.F. (ed.), Techniques of Biocompatibility Testing, Vol.II: p. 151 (1986).
6. Klinkmann, H., Wolf, H., Schmitt, E.: Definition of biocompatibility. Contrib. Nephrol. 37:70 (1984).
7. Craddock, P.R., Fehr, J., Dalmasso, A.P., Brigham, K.L., Jacob, H.S.: Hemodialysis leukopenia. Pulmonary vascular leucostasis resulting from complement activation by dialyzer cellophane membranes. J. Clin. Invest. 59:879 (1977).
8. Ivanovich, P., Chenoweth, D.E., Schmidt, R., Klinkmann, H., Boxer, L.A., Jacob, H.S., Hammerschmidt, D.E.: Symptoms and activation of granulocytes and complement with two dialysis membranes. Kidney Int. 24:758 (1983).
9. Chenoweth, D.E.: Biocompatibility of hemodialysis membranes. Evaluation with C3a anaphylatoxin radioimmunoassays. Am. Soc. Artif. Intern. Organs J. 7:44 (1984).
10. Hakim, R.M., Fearon, D.T., Lazarus, J.M.: Biocompatibility of dialysis membranes: effects of chronic complement activation. Kidney Int. 26:194 (1984).
11. Wegmüller, E., Montandon, A., Nydegger, U., Desceudres, D.: Biocompatibility of different hemodialysis membranes: activation of complement and leukopenia. Int. J. Artif. Organs 9:85 (1986).
12. Chenoweth, D.E., Cheung, A.L., Ward, D.M., Henderson, L.W.: Anaphylatoxin formation during hemodialysis: effects of two different dialyzer membranes. Kidney Int. 24:764 (1983).
13. Bingel, M., Lonnemann, G., Shaldon, S., Koch, K.M., Dinarello, C.A.: Human interleukin-1 production during hemodialysis. Nephron 43:161 (1986).
14. Cooper, N.R.: The complement system. In: Fundenberg, H.W., Sites, D.P., Caldwell, J.L., Wells, J.V., (eds.), Basic and Clinical Immunology, Chapter 6, Lange Medical Publications, Los Altos, CA (1976).
15. Rudy, S., Gigli, L., Austen, K.F.: The complement system of man. New Engl. J. Med. 287:489, 545, 592, 642 (1972).
16. Henderson, L.W., Cheung, A.K., Chenoweth, D.E.: Choosing a membrane. Am. J. Kidney Dis. 3:5 (1983).
17. Hoenich, N.A., Johnston, S.R.D., Woffindin, C., Kerr, D.N.S.: Hemodialyzers leucopenia: the role of membrane type and re-use. Contr. Nephrol. 37:120 (1984).
18. Falkenhagen, D., Bosch, T., Brown, G.S., Schmidt, R., Holtz, M., Bauermeister, U., Gurland, H., Klinkmann, H.: A clinical study on different cellulosic dialysis membranes. Nephrol. Dial. Transplant. 2:537 (1985).
19. Bosch, T., Schmidt, B., Samtleben, W., Gurland, H.J.: Biocompatibility and clinical performance of a new modified cellulose membranes. Clin. Nephrol. 26 (Suppl. 1):S22 (1986).
20. Klinkmann, H.: Clinical Relevance of Biocompatibility in Hemodialysis. "Verhandelingen van de Koningklijke Academie voor Geneeskunde van Belgie", XLIX 1:59 (1987).

21. Aljama, P., Bird, D.A.E., Ward, M.K., Feest, T.G., Walker, W., Tanboga, H.: Hemodialysis-induced leucopenia and activation of complement. Effects of different membranes. Proc. Eur. Dial. Transplant. Assoc. 15:144 (1978).

22. Jacob, A.J., Gavellas, G., Zarco, R., Perez, G., Bourgoignie, J.J.: Leucopenia, hypoxia and complement function with different hemodialysis membranes. Kidney Int. 18:505 (1980).

23. Jorstadt, S., Smeby, L.C., Balstad, T., Wideroe, T.-E.: Generation and removal of anaphylatoxins during hemofiltration with five different membranes. Blood Purif. 6:325 (1988).

24. Shaldon, S., Deschodt, G., Branger, B., Granolleras, G., Baldamus, C.A., Koch, K.M., Lysaght, M.J., Dinarello, C.A.: Hemodialysis hypotension: The interleukin hypothesis restated. Proc. Eur. Dial. Transplant. Ass. 22:229 (1985).

25. Lonnemann, G., Koch, K.M., Shaldon, S., Dinarello, C.A.: Plasma interleukin-1 activity in humans undergoing hemodialysis with regenerated cellulosic membranes. Lymphokine Res. 6:63 (1987).

26. Dinarello, C.A.: Interleukin-1 - Its multiple biological effects and its association with hemodialysis. Blood Purif. 6:164 (1988).

27. Vanherweghem, J.L., Drukker, W., Schwarz, A.: Clinical significance of blood-device interaction in hemodialysis. A review. Int. J. Artif. Organs. 10:219 (1987).

28. Gejyo, R., Yamada, T., Oami, S., Nakagawa, Y., Kunimoto, T.,Kataoka, H., Sizuki, M., Hirasawa, Y., Shirahama, T., Cohen, A.S., Schmid, K.: A new form of amyloid protein associated with hemodialysis was identified as β_2-microglobulin. Biochem. Biophys. Res. Commun. 129:701 (1985).

29. Ritz, E., Bommer, J.: Beta-2-microglobulin-derived amyloid - problems and perspectives. Blood Purif. 6:61 (1988).

30. Floege, J., Granolleras, C., Koch, K.M., Shaldon, S.: Which membrane? Should beta-2-microglobulin decide on the choice of today's hemodialysis membrane? Nephron 50:177 (1988).

31. Schmidt, H.: Staphylococcus saprophyticus als Erreger von Harnwegsinfektionen. B-Promotion, Rostock (1988).

TREATMENT OF URAEMIC ANAEMIA WITH RECOMBINANT HUMAN ERYTHROPOIETIN

Claudio Ponticelli, Stefano Casati,
Mariarosaria Campise

Divisione di Nefrologia, IRCCS Ospedale
Maggiore, Milan, Italy

Several factors have been involved in the pathogenesis of uraemic anaemia: inhibition of erythropoiesis and hyperhaemolysis to uraemic toxins (1); iron deficiency due to blood losses in the extracorporeal circuit (2); severe hyperparathyroidism with osteitis fibrosa (3); abnormally high concentrations of aluminium (4). However, there is general agreement that the main cause of uraemic anaemia is the insufficient production of erythropoietin from the diseased kidneys (5).

Recently, human erythropoietin has been isolated from the urine of patients with aplastic anaemia, characterized and cloned in cultured mammalian cells. Then, recombinant human erythropoietin (rHuEPO) has been made available in sufficient amounts to start pilot studies in order to assess rHuEPO efficacy and safety in chronic haemodialysis patients (6-8).

Five multicentre studies with large number of patients have confirmed the effectiveness of rHuEPO in uraemic anaemia. Entrance criteria, common to all trials, required stable clinical conditions, haematocrit lower than 30 % with no additional cause for anaemia than uraemia. In the first European trial (9) 150 patients were enrolled , 9 of whom were then excluded for different reasons. All 141 patients had an individual haemoglobin (Hb) increase of at least 2 g/dl. In most of them (93 %) the response was obtained with a dose of 192 units/kg b. w. three times a week. Four patients who did not respond were found to have iron deficiency and low serum ferritin levels. Full correction of anaemia, arbitrarily defined as Hb between 10-12 g/dl, could be maintained by a weekly dose of 200 units/kg divided into 2-3 applications. In a second still ongoing European trial 43 transfusion dependent patients were studied. The starting dose was 100 units/kg 3 times a week. Full response was observed in all the patients within

12-20 weeks. No patient required blood transfusions after rHuEPO treatment was started. In a cooperative American multicentre trial (10) 247 haemodialysis patients were treated with 150-200 units/kg i.v. 3 times a week. All but 6 patients responded with a mean haematocrit increase from 22.9 % to 33.5 %. Blood transfusions were required by 127 patients before rHuEPO was started, but only 3 of them required further blood transfusions during rHuEPO therapy. In a multicentre German study 92 haemodialysis patients were studied. In this study rHuEPO doses ranged 40-120 units/kg three times a week. The median increment of haematocrit per week was dose dependent and ranged 0.69-1.55 %. The rise in reticulocyte count was greater in patients receiving three times weekly 80 or 120 units/kg than in patients receiving only 40 units/kg. Reticulocyte count reached its maximum after 3-4 weeks in all groups, but the maximal level remained much lower in the group receiving only 40 units/kg three times a week (11). Finally, in a multicentre Japanese study (12) 66 patients were treated with rHuEPO at doses ranging 50-200 units/kg 3 times a week. All patients responded with haematocrit rising from 19.8 ± 2.3 % to 30.2 ± 4.9 % after 12 weeks of treatment. Of the 66 patients considered, 32 required a total of 206 units of blood during the 3 months pretreatment controlled period. Only 34 blood units had to be administered to 17 patients after rHuEPO therapy.

In all these multicentre studies iron and ferritin decreased significantly during rHuEPO therapy, due to a hypersynthesis of Hb. As a consequence functional iron deficiency may develop in patients with normal iron stores. The decreased availability of iron can interfere with the response to rHuEPO. Therefore the iron stores should be checked during rHuEPO therapy and iron supplementation should be given when needed at doses able to maintain the percent transferrin saturation above 20 and serum ferritin concentrations around 100 ng/ml.

Aluminium is thought to interfere with a normal marrow response to rHuEPO. The body pool of this trace element is frequently increased in haemodialysis patients and it appears to interfere with the release of the transferrin bound iron to the erythroid cell (14). A negative correlation was found between the levels of plasma aluminium after a desferrioxamine test and the doses of rHuEPO required to increase Hb by 2 g/dl (8). These data confirm that aluminium intoxication can alter the bone marrow sensitivity to rHuEPO but also indicate that higher doses of rHuEPO can correct anaemia also in aluminium intoxicated patients. On the contrary, no relationship could be observed between parathyroid hormone serum levels and response to rHuEPO (8,14).

Besides iron and aluminium, also the occurrence of adverse events during rHuEPO can reprecipitate anaemia. In fact, it has been reported that surgery (13) and infections (15) are accompanied by reduction of haemoglobin levels despite rHuEPO administration. After resolution of these complications reticulocytosis and erythropoiesis resumed, though requiring many weeks before the previous haemoglobin levels were achieved. This would suggest that anaemia due to inflammatory causes is independent of erythropoietin administration or secretion (15).

ADVANTAGES OF CORRECTION OF ANAEMIA

Increased appetite, improved sleep, relief from Raynaud's phenomenon, less depression, increased hair growth, improved sexual function and return to menstrual cycles have been widely reported (15,16). Moreover, increase in energy and exercise tolerance after correction of anaemia have been referred by many patients and reported as increased oxygen uptake at the anaerobic threshold (from 13.7 ± 2 to 19.1 ± 3.4 ml/kg/min; $p < 0.01$) and peak peripheral oxygen uptake at subjective exhaustion (from 16 ± 3.4 to 23.2 ± 8.2 ml/kg/min; $p < 0.02$) (17).

The reduction of iron and iron stores observed in the majority of the rHuEPO treated patients can be considered of beneficial in those patients who present an iron overload caused by blood transfusions or excessive iron supplementation. A mean decrease of ferritin of approximately 90 ng/ml/week has been observed in dialysis patients receiving 150 units/kg 3 times a week (6).

It has been reported (6,18-21) that correction of anaemia with rHuEPO can correct the cardiac dilation so frequently observed in severely anaemic dialysis patients. Moreover, after Hb levels had improved, both clinical and electrocardiographic signs of angina and ischaemia had improved. Cardiac performances, measured as cardiac output and ejection fraction, improved after rHuEPO therapy (22). A possible disadvantage might be the reported increase in plasma natriuretic peptide following full correction of anaemia which can be considered as an indicator of a raised blood volume. This could lead in the long term to an increased intraatrial pressure (20).

It is well known that uraemic patients have a defect of primary haemostasis expressed as a prolonged skin bleeding time and altered platelet aggregation and adhesion to vessel wall (23). It has also been demonstrated the important role of anaemia in the pathogenesis of this defect, which can be temporarily reversed by blood transfusions (24). The behaviour of haemostasis have been studied in a group of patients treated with rHuEPO. The progressive rise in haematocrit induced by rHuEPO was paralleled by a significant shortening of the bleeding time from a median of more than 30 minutes to 8 minutes (25). Moreover, the changes in blood rheology also influenced platelet adhesion to subendothelium (25). The improvement in the haemostatic defect during rHuEPO occurred soon after the start of rHuEPO to haematocrit values of about 30 %. Changes in red cells rheology can be considered as the most important cause for this improvement, although a direct role for rHuEPO in promoting an effect on megakariocytes cannot be excluded (26).

SIDE EFFECTS

No allergic reactions to rHuEPO have been reported so far. Only exceptionally rHuEPO therapy had to be discontinued either because of joint pain or headache after infusion (27). In some cases rHuEPO had to be discontinued because of the development of severe hypertension. The prevalence of hypertension associated with rHuEPO therapy ranged about 20 % in the first European trial (9) and about 32 % in the American multicentre study (10). Worsening of blood pressure was reported more frequently in previously hypertensive patients (8). In some cases the rise in blood pressure was accompanied by grand mal seizures (7,10,28-30). The causes of hypertension induced by rHuEPO have not been completely elucidated, but the increase in blood viscosity (31) and peripheral resistances (32) induced by the correction of anaemia may play an important role. Many factors may contribute to the rise in peripheral resistances: changes in plasma catecholamines, reversal of the vasodilating effect of anaemia (33), increased binding by haemoglobin of nitric oxide a potent natural vasodilating agent (34), increased blood viscosity (35).

Following the correction of anaemia an increased dosage of heparin was commonly required to avoid clotting of the extracorporeal circuit during the dialysis treatment. Thrombosis of the vascular access was reported in many patients: 14 of 150 of the first European trial suffered from this complication (9). In the American multicentre study thrombosis of the arterio-venous fistula was observed in only 4 of 247 patients (10) and in the German study this problem was reported in 5 of 92 patients (27). This increased tendency to clot during rHuEPO therapy is correlated with the correction of the haemostatic defect induced by the rise of the haematocrit (25).

The correction of anaemia, through the increased blood viscosity and clotting tendency may theoretically induce a reduction of dialysis efficiency by lowering the effective plasma flow and by favouring clotting in the dialyzers. Controversy still exists among authors concerning this point: a 13 % rise of predialysis serum creatinine has been observed during rHuEPO treatment in the pilot study of Eschbach (6). Other studies did not evidentiate any change in predialysis urea and creatinine levels after rHuEPO treatment (8,16,35). Improvement in predialysis serum urea levels have been even reported in patients treated with high efficiency haemodialysis (36).

Despite an unchanged dialysis efficiency, a tendency to hyperkalaemia has been reported in several studies (6,8). Cationic exchange resins had to be given to many patients in order to correct hyperkalaemia. Hyperkalaemia was attributed to the increased intake of potassium with food and to the increased release of potassium into the plasma from the greater number of red cells which are haemolyzed daily.

CONCLUSIONS

In most uraemic patients anaemia can fully corrected by rHuEPO. As shown, many factors can influence the response to the treatment requiring an almost individual dosage of the drug. The quality of life of haemodialysis patients under rHuEPO treatment significantly improved and many symptoms reversed. Hypertension and thrombotic complications seem to have a higher incidence in the rHuEPO treated patients. These complications may be minimized by giving rHuEPO in small doses with small increments to avoid a too rapid correction and allowing an adequate resetting of the homeostatic mechanism to the new conditions provoked. A partial correction of anaemia (haemoglobin around 10 g/dl) while sufficient to reverse many symptoms may prevent or reduce the risk of major complications.

REFERENCES

1. Markson, J.L., Renniec, J.B.: The anaemia of chronic renal insufficiency. Scott. Med. J. 1:320 (1970)
2. Loge, J.P., Lange, R.D., Moore, C.V.: Characterization of the anemia associated with chronic renal insufficiency. Am. J. Med. 24:4 (1958).
3. Weinberg, S.G., Lubin, A., Wiener, S., Deoras, M.P., Ghose, M.K., Kogelmann, R.C.: Myelofibrosis and renal osteodystrophy. Am. J. Med. 63: 755 (1977).
4. Kaiser, L., Schwartz, K.A.: Aluminium induced anaemia. Am. J. Kidney Dis. 6:348 (1985).
5. Eschbach, J.W., Adamson, J.W.: Anaemia of end stage renal disease. Kidney Int. 28:1 (1985).
6. Eschbach, J.W., Egrie, J.C., Downing, M.R., Browne, J.K., Adamson, J.W.: Correction of anaemia of end stage renal disease with recombinant human erythropoietin. N. Engl. J. Med. 316:73 (1987).
7. Winearls, C.G., Oliver, D.O., Pippard, M.J., Reid, C., Downing, M.R., Cotes, P.M.: Effect of human erythropoietin derived from recombinant DNA on the anaemia of patients maintained by chronic haemodialysis. Lancet 2:1175 (1986).
8. Casati, S., Passerini, P., Campise, M., Graziani, G., Cesana, B., Perisic, M., Ponticelli, C.: Benefits and risks of protracted treatment with human recombinant erythropoietin in patients having haemodialysis. Brit. Med. J. 4:1017 (1987).
9. Sundal, E., Bariety, J., Blumberg, A., Bommer, J., Canaud, B., Danielson, B., Kreis, H., Lamperi, S., Michielsen, P., Rhyner, K., Ponticelli, C., Schaefer, R.M., Verbeelen, D., Zehnder, C., Kaeser, U.: Correction of the anaemia of chronic renal failure with recombinant human erythropoietin: results from a multicentre study in 150 haemotransfusion dependent patients (submitted for publication).
10. Eschbach, J.W., Adamson, J.W.: Correction of the anemia of hemodialysis patients with recombinant human erythropoietin. Results of a multicentre study. Kidney Int. 33:189 (1988).
11. Bommer, J., Kugel, M., Schoeppe, W., Brunkhorst, R., Samtleben, W., Bramsiepe, W., Scigalla, P.: Dose related effects of recombinant human erythropoietin on

erythropoiesis. Results of a multicentre trial in patients with end-stage renal disease. Contr. Nephrol. Vol. 66, p 85, Karger, Basel, (1988).

12. Akizawa, T., Koshikawa, S., Takaku, F., Urabe, A., Akiyama, N., Mimura, N., Otsubo, O., Nihei, H., Suzuki, Y., Kawaguchi, Y., Ota, K., Kubo, K., Marumo, F., Maeda, T.: Clinical effect of recombinant human erythropoietin on anemia associated with chronic renal failure. A multi institutional study in Japan. Int. J. Artif. Organs. 11: 343 (1988).

13. Eschbach, J.W., Adamson, J.W.: Recombinant human erythropoietin: Implications for nephrology. Am. J. Kidney Dis. 11:203 (1988).

14. Hampl, H., Riedel, E., Wendel, G., Stabell U., Kessel, M.: Influence of parathyroid hormone on exogenous erythropoietin stimulated erythropoiesis in hemodialysis patients. Kidney Int. 33:224 (1988).

15. Winearls, C.G.: Use of erythropoietin in patients with end-stage renal disease. Royal Soc. Med. 1:2 (1988).

16. Bommer, J., Alexiou, C., Müller-Bühl, U., Eifert, J., Ritz, E.: Recombinant human erythropoietin therapy in hemodialysis patients. Dose determination and clinical experience. Nephrol. Dial. Transpl. 2:23 (1987).

17. Mayer, G., Thum, J. Cada, E.M., Stummvoll, H.K., Graf, H.: Working capacity is increased following recombinant human erythropoietin treatment. Kidney Int. 34:525 (1988).

18. Grützmacher, P., Bergmann M., Löw, I., Schoeppe, W.: Cardiac changes in haemodialysis patients treated by recombinant human erythropoietin. Int. Soc. Blood Purification, Vicenza June, Abstr. 36 (1988).

19. London, G.M., Zins, B., Naret, C., Pannier, B., Berthelot, J.M., Peterlongo, F., Drueke, T., Jacquot, C.: Hemodynamic changes in haemodialysis patients in response to recombinant erythropoietin. EDTA-ERA Madrid, Abstr. 211 (1988).

20. Kühn, K., Talartschik, H., Koch, K.M., Eisenhauer, T., Nonnast-Daniel, B., Scheler, F., Brunkhorst, R., Reimers, E.: Plasma atrial natriuretic peptide levels after partial correction of renal anemia by recombinant human erythropoietin. EDTA-ERA Madrid, Abstr. 210 (1988).

21. Mangiarotti, R., Pierini, A., Casati, S., Passerini, P., Ambroso, G.C., Pini, C., Graziani, G.: Modificazioni della funzionalità cardiaca nell'emodializzato in trattamento con eritropoietina. Nefrologia, Acta Medica, Roma 419 (1987).

22. Paganini, E., Thomas, T., Fouad, F., Garcia, J., Bravo, E.: The correction of anemia in hemodialysis patients using recombinant human erythropoietin: hemodynamic effects. Kidney Int. 33:204 (1988).

23. Deykin, D.: Uremic bleeding. Kidney Int. 24:698 (1983).

24. Livio, M., Marchesi, D., Remuzzi, G., Gotti, E., Mecca, G., DeGaetano, G.: Uraemic bleeding: role of anemia and beneficial effect of red-cell transfusions. Lancet 2:1013 (1982).

25. Moia, M., Vizzotto, L., Cattaneo, M., Mannucci, P.M., Casati, S., Ponticelli, C.: Improvement in the haemostatic defect of uraemia after treatment with recombinant human erythropoietin. Lancet 2:1227 (1987).

26. Ishibashi, T., Koziol, J.A., Burstein, S.A.: Human recombinant erythropoietin promotes differentiation of murine megakaryocytes in vitro. J. Clin. Invest. 79: 286 (1987).

27. Grützmacher, P., Bergmann, M., Nattermann, U., Weinreich, T., Reimers, E., Pollak, M.: Beneficial and adverse effects of correction of anaemia by recombinant human erythropoietin in patients on maintenance haemodialysis. Contr. Nephrol. Vol. 66, p 104, Karger, Basel, (1988).

28. Jacquot, C., Ferragu-Haguet, M., Lefebvre, A., Berthelot, J.M., Peterlongo, F., Castaigne, J.P.: Recombinant human erythropoietin and blood pressure. Lancet 2:1083 (1987).

29. Tomson, C.R.V., Venning, M.C., Ward, M.K.: Blood pressure and erythropoietin. Lancet 1:351 (1988).

30. Edmunds, M.S., Walls, J.: Blood pressure and erythropoietin. Lancet 1:352 (1988).

31. Neff, M.S., Kim, K.E., Persoff, M., Onesti, G., Swartz, C.: Haemodynamics of uraemic anaemia. Circulation 43:876 (1971).

32. Capelli, J.P., Kasparian, H.: Cardiac work demands and left ventricular function in end-stage renal disease. Ann. Intern. Med. 86:261 (1977).

33. Colemann, T.G.: Hemodynamics of uremic anemia. Circulation 45:510 (1972).

34. Martin, J., Moncada, S.: Blood pressure, erythropoietin and nitric oxide. Lancet 1:644 (1988).

35. Schaefer, R.M., Kuerner, B., Zech, M., Denninger, G., Borneff, C., Heidland, A.: Treatment of the anemia of hemodialysis patients with recombinant human erythropoietin. Int. J. Artif. Organs 11:249 (1988).

36. Stivelmann, J., van Wick, D., Kirlin, D., Ogden, D.: Use of recombinant erythropoietin with high flux dialysis does not worsen azotemia or shorten access survival. Kidney Int. 33:239 (1988).

ENDOCRINE ABNORMALITIES IN PATIENTS WITH ENDSTAGE RENAL FAILURE*

F. Kokot[1], A. Wiecek[1], W. Grzeszczak[1],
J. Klepacka[2], M. Klin[1], M. Lao[2]

[1] Department of Nephrology Silesian School of
Medicine, Katowice, and
[2] Institute of Transplantation, Medical Academy
of Warsaw

Renal failure is associated with major endocrine abnormalities. These abnormalities seem to be caused not only by the reduced excretory and biodegradatory functions of the diseased kidneys, but also as consequence of the adaptive mechanism to renal failure and the accumulation of uraemic toxins. Additionally, nutritional factors and medical treatment may influence the type and magnitude of endocrine abnormalities noted in renal failure patients [1,2].

In this paper we will present only a) selected topics concerning the importance of opioid receptors in the pathogenesis of endocrine abnormalities and b) the influence of erythropoietin treatment on hormonal alterations in patients with endstage renal failure.

A. Importance of opioid receptors in the pathogenesis of endocrine alterations

Several lines of evidence suggest a role of opioids in the regulation of endocrine function. First, opioid peptide precursors have been found in different endocrine organs both in health and disease[3]. Second, opioid receptors have been identified in the cell membranes of endocrine organs[4,5]. Third, administration of exogenous opioids alters the function of endocrine glands[5]. Fourth, endogenous opioid peptides, acting as central neurotransmitters, may indirectly influence endocrine function[6].

*Supported in part by the Polish Ministry of Health and Welfare, MZ XIII

Theoretically three approaches might be used to investigate the role of opioids in renal failure: 1) measurement of plasma levels of opioid peptides and their relationship to concomitant endocrine abnormalities;
2) assessment of endocrine organ function in patients with
renal failure before and after opioid receptors blockade,
and 3) estimation of opioids within endocrine organs by im-
munohistochemistry. In clinical practice, only the first
two methods are feasible in patients. We chose the second
one using the opioid receptor antagonist naloxone. This antagonist, if used in an appropriate dose, can differen-
tiate opioid effects mediated by opioid receptors from
those realized by other pathways.

In patients presented in this paper secretion of individual hormones were studied twice under stimulatory or
inhibitory conditions, first without naloxone and a second
time, after intravenous administration of 2 mg of this
drug. Methodological details are given in our previous
studies[7].

a) PTH and Calcitonin

The secretion of PTH and calcitonin was assessed
during an i. v. calcium infusion[8]. In uraemic patients
(CRF) the mean increase of serum calcium level was 0.84
mmol/l before naloxone and 1.40 ± 0.14 mmol/l after opioid
receptor blockade (p < 0.05) compared with control values
of 0.51 ± 0.1 and 0.74 ± 0.1 mmol/l, respectively
(p < 0.05).

Before naloxone, calcium infusion was followed by significant declines in serum PTH levels (-1.16 ± 0.25 ng/ml
in uraemic patients and -0.31 ± 0.04 ng/ml in normals,
p < 0.005) and elevations in plasma calcitonin concentrations (+389 ± 99.4 pg/ml in CRF and 316 ± 63.7 pg/ml in
normal, the difference is statistically not significant).
Patients with CRF differed from normal subjects, in
response to calcium infusion after blockade of opioid receptors. Suppression of PTH secretion was blunted in CRF
(= 0.0 ± 0.16 ng/ml) but normal (-0.20 ± 0.06 ng/ml) in
healthy subjects, while calcitonin secretion was significantly diminished (= +115 ± 81.7 pg/ml) in uraemic patients and unchanged (= +378 ± 97 ng/ml) in normals.

b) Insulin and glucagon

The influence of naloxone on insulin and glucagon
secretion was studied in patients after an oral glucose
load[9]. In uraemic patients the mean increase in blood
glucose level after an oral glucose load was 3.70 ± 0.42
mmol/l without naloxone and 2.36 ± 0.09 mmol/l after administration of this drug (p < 0.05). The respective values
obtained in controls were 2.87 ± 0.28 and 2.18 ± 0.18 mmol/l
(p < 0.05). Before opioid receptor blockade the mean
increase of plasma insulin was 17.4 ± 4.2 µU/ml in CRF and
18.4 ± 4.6 µU/ml in controls (the difference is statistically not significant). Naloxone administration was
followed by an enhanced responsiveness of insulin secretion
both in uraemic patients and controls. This increased

responsiveness was significantly (p < 0.05) more marked in patients (= 42.5 ± 7.9 µU/ml) than in normals (= 24.4 ± 4.2 µU/ml).

A significant increase in plasma glucagon level occured during the second period of the oral glucose tolerance test (performed without naloxone) both in CRF (mean increase 120 ± 38 pg/ml) and in controls (mean increase 70 ± 14 pg/ml). Naloxone almost completely blunted the increase in glucagon in both examined groups. Suppression of plasma glucagon was significantly (p < 0.001) greater in uraemic patients (= mean change -87 ± 10 pg/ml) than in normals (7.8 ± 16 pg/ml).

From the above presented result it follows that existence of hyperendorphinism in chronic uraemia is highly likely. The question arises, whether this is a purposeful compensatory mechanism involved in improving the disturbed internal environment or a factor contributing to the uraemic state?

The results of our naloxone studies of PTH and CT secretion in uraemic patients suggest, that hyperendorphinism is a purposeful compensatory mechanism, which makes cells of the parathyroid glands and thyroid C cells more sensitive to changes in plasma calcium levels counteracting secondary hyperparathyroidism. To the extent that PTH is incriminated as an uraemic toxin[10] its suppression by endogenous opioids could have beneficial effects not only on the metabolism of calcium and phosphate but also on the function of different organs. Harmful "side-effects" of this compensatory hyperendorphinism in chronic renal failure patients are the impairment of the glucose tolerance evoked by enhanced glucagon and suppressed insulin secretion.

It may be postulated that hyperendorphinism in uraemic patients may be regarded both as a primary beneficial compensatory mechanism counteracting disturbances of the internal environment, while causing secondary harmful side effects which contribute to the uraemic state.

B. Influence of erythropoietin treatment on endocrine alterations in haemodialyzed patients with endstage renal failure

Recombinant human erythropoietin (rh-E, Cilag) was administered to haemodialyzed patients with endstage renal failure for 12-13 weeks. The mean dose of rh-E was 75 units/kg b. w. administered i. v. 3 times per week immediately after a haemodialysis session. All hormones were estimated in blood samples withdrawn in the morning from fasting patients. All hormones were estimated by radioimmunoassay[11] before and after 12-13 weeks of rh-E treatment. After rh-E treatment the haemoglobin level rose from 4.47 ± 0.18 to 6.67 ± 0.15 mmol/l while the haematocrit value from 23 ± 0.89 % to 34.6 ± 0.74 %, respectively.

Table 1. Influence of recombinant human erythropoietin
treatment for 12-13 weeks on basal plasma levels
of somatotropin (HGH), ACTH, prolactin (PRL),
vasopressin (AVP), insulin (IRI) and glucagon
(IRG) in haemodialyzed patients with chronic renal failure (CRF). Normal values of the individual hormones obtained in healthy subjects
are also enlisted. N - number of subjects.
Means ± SEM.

	Patients with CRF before	after	Healthy subjects
		treatment	
HGH ng/ml	9.52 ± 1.14	4.81 ± 0.66	3.55 ± 0.53
N	11	11	14
ACTH pg/ml	58.80 ± 4.40	13.20 ± 2.15	23.60 ± 1.86
N	5	5	15
PRL ng/ml	36.78 ± 4.65	12.88 ± 2.62	12.10 ± 1.60
N	11	11	12
AVP pg/ml	6.40 ± 1.70	6.24 ± 1.32	2.11 ± 0.16
N	5	5	10
IRI mU/l	19.80 ± 3.56	29.20 ± 3.35	8.60 ± 1.20
N	11	11	15
IRG ng/l	256.00 ± 61.42	114.00 ± 41.98	115.00 ± 17.00
N	5	5	15

a) Pituitary hormones (somatotropin - STH, corticotrophin -
ACTH, prolactin - Pro, vasopressin - AVP)

Before rh-E treatment basal STH, ACTH, Pro and AVP
plasma levels in uraemic patients were significantly higher
than in normals (table 1.). After rh-E treatment plasma levels of STH, ACTH and Pro decreased significantly and were
in the normal range, while plasma AVP concentration remained unchanged.

b)   Pancreatic hormones (insulin - IRI, glucagon - IRG)

As can be seen in table 1 uraemic patients showed
significantly elevated plasma levels of IRI and IRG as
compared with normals. After rh-E treatment plasma IRI le-

vels in uraemic patients rose significantly while IRG
concentrations declined to the normal range.

c) Atrial natriuretic peptide (ANP), plasma renin activity (PRA), aldosterone (Ald) and cortisol (C)

As shown in table 2 before rh-E treatment basal
values of ANP, PRA and Ald were significantly elevated as
compared with normals, while plasma cortisol levels were in
the normal range. After rh-E treatment a significant
decline of PRA, Ald and C was noticed. In contrast to
these hormones rh-E treatment was followed by a significant
increase of plasma ANP level.

d) Parathyroid hormone (PTH) and calcitonin (CT)

As can be seen in table 2 uraemic patients showed
significantly higher plasma levels of PTH and CT than normals. No influence of rh-E treatment on plasma concentrations of the above mentioned two hormones was observed.

Table 2. Influence of rh-erythropoietin treatment for
12-13 weeks on basal plasma levels of atrial
natriuretic peptide (ANF), plasma renin activity (PRA), aldosterone (Ald), cortisol (C),
parathyroid hormone (PTH) and calcitonin (CT) in
haemodialyzed patients with chronic renal failure.
Normal values of the individual hormones obtained
in healthy subjects are also enlisted. N - number
of subjects. Means ± SEM.

		Patients with CRF before after treatment		Healthy subjects
ANP pg/ml	N	± 159.20 12.73 5	± 254.60 38.03 5	± 74.10 7.10 10
PRA ng/ml	N	± 5.39 0.76 11	± 3.26 0.61 11	± 2.78 0.18 10
Ald ng/dl	N	± 18.34 4.15 11	± 13.04 1.14 11	± 9.76 0.70 10
C µg/dl	N	± 13.24 2.07 5	± 7.88 1.18 5	± 12.40 1.80 12
PTH ng/ml	N	± 1.60 0.41 5	± 2.08 0.31 5	± 0.62 0.05 13
CT ng/ml	N	109.00 20.39 5	149.00 40.93 5	21.77 3.29 13

As shown in table 1 and 2 rh-E treatment exhibits a marked influence on function of endocrine organs. While STH, ACTH, Pro, IRG, PRA, Ald and C secretion seems to be suppressed by rh-E treatment, IRI and ANP secretion are stimulated. Finally rh-E treatment did not influence significantly plasma levels of AVP, PTH and CT. The pathogenesis and clinical importance of the rh-E induced hormonal alterations remain to be elucidated. It seems very likely that suppression of PRA and Ald and stimulation of ANP secretion were caused by an increase of circulating blood volume (as suggested by Kühn[12]) evoked by rh-E induced increase of erythropoiesis. As well known hypervolaemia is suppressing renin and aldosterone secretion while ANP release is stimulated. As hypervolaemia is also suppressing AVP secretion a decrease of plasma AVP could also be expected. Contrary to these expectations rh-E treatment did not influence significantly plasma AVP levels. Thus it seems, that abnormal AVP secretion in uraemic patients is not corrected by rh-E treatment.

As shown in this study rh-E treatment evoked an unexpected influence on plasma levels of STH, ACTH, Pro, IRI and IRG. It remains to be elucidated whether this effect of rh-E is a consequence of corrected anaemia and improved tissue perfusion or reflects a specific effect of rh-E itself. As already reported by Schaefer et al.[13] and confirmed in this study, rh-E treatment was followed by significant decline of plasma Pro levels. This decline could be involved in the improvement of sexual function in rh-E treated patients. As already reported by Bommer et al.[14] suppression of Pro may improve sexual activity in uraemic patients.

The pathophysiological relevance of rh-E treatment on IRI, IRG and STH secretion remains to be clarified. It seems very likely that improvement of carbohydrate tolerance in rh-E treated patients (unpublished own observations) are at least in part related to the stimulatory effect of rh-E on IRI secretion and to the suppressive effect of this hormone on STH and IRG release.

Data presented in this study suggest that most endocrine abnormalities in uraemic patients are not or only in part consequence of impaired renal excretion and (or) biodegradation of hormones. Thus reconsideration of the pathogenesis of endocrine abnormalities in uraemic patients seems to be mandatory.

Summary

Data presented in this study suggest existence of hyperendorphinism in uraemic patients. This hyperendorphinism may be regarded both as a primary beneficial compensatory mechanism counteracting disturbances of the internal environment, while causing secondary harmful side effects, which contribute to the uraemic state.

Erythropoietin treatment of uraemic, haemodialyzed patients is followed by marked endocrine alterations (sup-

pression of plasma levels of STH, ACTH, prolactin, glucagon, aldosterone, cortisol and plasma renin activity, elevation of plasma insulin and atrial natriuretic levels,
lack of influence on plasma PTH, CT and AVP). It remains
to be clarified whether the erythropoietin induced endocrine alterations are due to correction of the existing
anaemia or reflect a specific effect of this hormone.

References

1. Osten, B., Kokot F. and Klinkmann, H.: Endokrinolo-
    gische Störungen bei chronischer Niereninsuffizienz
    und bei Dauerdialysebehandlung. Teil 1, Renale
    Hormone-Hypophyse. Dtsch. Gesundh.-Wesen 37:2113
    (1982).
2. Osten, B., Kokot, F. and Klinkmann, H.: Endokrinolo-
    gische Störungen bei chronischer Niereninsuffizienz
    bei Dauerdialysebehandlung. Teil 2, Schilddrüse-
    Nebenschilddrüse-Gastrin-Pancreas-Nebenniere-Gonaden.
    Dtsch. Gesundh.-Wesen 37:2196 (1982).
3. Bostwick, D.G., Null, W.E., Holmes, D., Weber, E.,
    Barchas, J.D. and Bensch, K.G.: Expression of opioid
    peptides in tumors. N. Engl. J. Med. 317:1439 (1987).
4. Kriger, D.T.: Endorphins and enkephalins, in "Yearbook
    Medical Publishers", Chicago (1982).
5. Pfeiffer, A. and Herz, A.: Endocrine actions of
    opioids. Horm. Metabol. Res. 16:386 (1984).
6. Clement-Jones, V. and Besser, G.M.: Clinical perspec-
    tives in opioid peptides. Br. Med. Bul. 39:95 (1984).
7. Grzeszczak, W., Kokot, F. and Dulawa, J.: Effects of
    naloxone administration on endocrine abnormalities in
    chronic renal failure. Am. J. Nephrol. 7:93 (1987).
8. Grzeszczak, W., Kokot, F. and Dulawa, J.: Einfluss von
    Naloxone auf die Parathormon- und Calcitoninsekretion
    bei Kranken mit akuter und chronischer Niereninsuffi-
    zienz. Z. Klin. Med. 41:435 (1986).
9. Grzeszczak, W., Kokot, F. and Dulawa, J.: Wplyw
    naloksonu na sekrecje insuliny i glukagonu u chorych
    na ostra niewydolnosc nerek (Influence of naloxone on
    insulin and glucagon secretion in acute renal failu-
    re). Pol. Tyg. Lek. 41:331 (1986).
10. Massry, S.G.: Current status of the role of parathy-
    roid hormone in uremic toxicity. Contrib. Nephrol.
    49:1 (1985).
11. Kokot, F., Stupnicki, R.: "Metody radioimmunologiczne
    i radiokompetycyjne stosowane w klinice" (Radioimmuno-
    assay and radiocompetitive methods used in clinical
    practice). PZWL, Warszawa (1985).
12. Kühn, K., Talartschik, H., Koch, K.M., Eisenhauer, T.,
    Nonnast-Daniel, B., Scheler, Brunkhorst, R. and
    Reiner, E.: Plasma atrial natriuretic peptide after
    partial correction of renal anaemia by recombinant
    human erythropoietin. Nephrol. Dial. Transplant. 3:
    497 (1988) (Abstract).
13. Schaefer, R.M., Kokot, F. and Heidland, A.: Normali-
    zation of prolactin levels and improved sexual function
    in dialysis patients on erythropoietin. Nephrol. Dial.
    Transplant. 3:501 (1988) (Abstract).
14. Bommer, J., Del Pozo, E., Ritz, E. and Bommer, G.:
    Improved sexual function in male haemodialysis patients
    on bromocriptine. Lancet 2:496 (1979).

CARNITINE SUPPLEMENTATION IN UREMIA

Peter Fürst, Anne Glöggler, Claudia Rössle*

Institut für Biologische Chemie und Ernährungs-
wissenschaft, Universität Hohenheim
D-7000 Stuttgart 70, and *Laboratoire de
Nutrition, Hopital St. Pierre, B-1000 Bruxelles

BIOCHEMICAL CONSIDERATIONS

Biosynthesis

In humans, L-carnitine (L-(-)-3-hydroxy-4-trimethyl-
aminobutyrate, molecular weight 62 daltons) is synthesized
in the liver, kidney and brain from the two essential amino
acids lysine and methionine mediated by a multi-enzyme
system[1]. Four co-factors - vitamin C, niacin, vitamin B_6,
and iron - are required by the various enzymes[2,3]. The rare
amino acid N-6-trimethyllysine (TML) is formed by post-
translational methylation of lysine residues with S-adeno-
sylmethionine[4]. Once released by proteolytic action, it may
serve as a precursor for the endogenous biosynthesis of
carnitine[5]. TML is converted to L-carnitine via four en-
zymatic steps (hydroxylation, aldol cleavage, oxidation and
a second hydroxylation).

Carnitine functions

The transport of long-chain fatty acid esters to sites
of beta-oxidation in the mitochondrial matrix requires L-
carnitine[6]. The carnitine carrier system consists of
carnitine, carnitine-palmitoyl-transferase (CPT) I and II
and the carnitine-acylcarnitine-translocase. CPT I located
on the outer side of the inner mitochondrial membrane,
transferes activated long-chain acylresidues from acyl-CoA
to carnitine. The translocase shuttles acylcarnitine across
the mitochondrial membrane, where CPT II catalyses the
formation of acyl-CoA from free and acylcarnitine[7]. The
activated fatty acid can subsequently undergo beta-oxidation. Since the inner membrane of the mitochondria is
impermeable to long-chain fatty acids their transport into
the mitochondrial matrix is dependent upon adequate concentrations of carnitine.

It has been recognized that there is a role of carnitine in buffering the bound CoA to free CoA ratio[8,9].

Coenzyme A is an important intermediate in many metabolic
pathways. In conditions in which the major portion of the
coenzyme A is bound free CoA is not available for essential
metabolic reactions. Nevertheless, the acyl moiety of the
bound CoA can be transferred to carnitine by action of one
of the acylcarnitine transferases producing free CoA.

It is also largely accepted that carnitine may shuttle
acetyl groups from the mitochondria and the peroxisomes into the cytosol via the acetyl transferase reaction where
fatty acid synthesis takes place[10]. This modus of transport is indeed inexpensive, unlike to the citrate pathway
which requires ample amounts of ATP[8]. Therefore it has been
recently suggested that carnitine is similarly important
for the transport of the acyl groups (metabolic energy)
from one cell to another cell and into the appropriate cellular compartment. By modulating the tissue content of acyl-
CoA compounds which inhibit many enzyme activities carnitine
thus may regulate certain metabolic pathways[8,10].

CARNITINE STATUS IN CHRONIC UREMIA

Carnitine deficiency has been repeatedly claimed in the
state of chronic uremia[11,12]. There are numerous causes of
carnitine depletion in dialysis patients like carnitine loss
in dialysis fluid, low dietary intake of carnitine, reduced
carnitine absorption in gut, diminished liver synthesis and
ceased capacity to synthesize carnitine by the diseased
kidney[9].

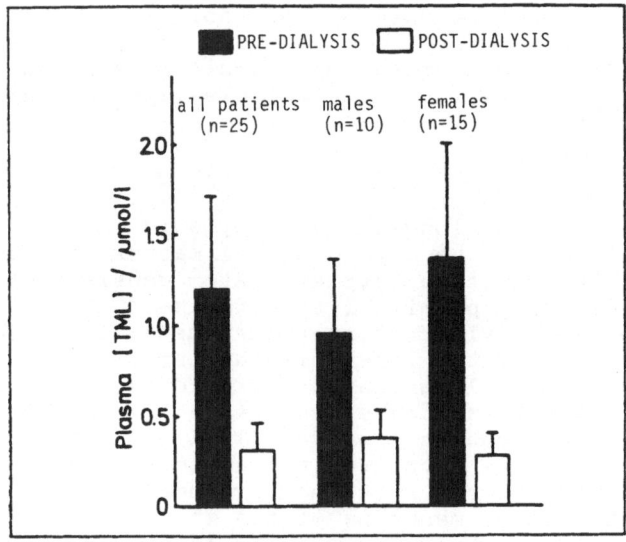

Fig. 1 Mean plasma-free TML concentrations in hemodialysis
patients determined prior to (shaded blocks) and immediately
after (open blocks) the dialysis treatment. Standard deviations are represented by the bars. Mean value of normal
persons: 0.290 ± 0.164 μmol/l (SD). From ref. 13.

TABLE 1

Serum total, free and esterified carnitine levels in hemodialysis patients compared to controls.

Carnitine fraction	Hemodialysis patients	Controls
μmol/l	n = 23	n = 20
Total carnitine (TC)	50 ± 4	46 ± 3
Free carnitine (FC)	32 ± 3*	38 ± 2
Short-chain acyl-carnitine (SCC)	17 ± 2	8 ± 1
Long-chain acyl-carnitine (LCC)	1.2 ± 0.2*	0.6 ± 0.1
Ratio of AC/FC	0.6 ± 0.07**	0.2 ± 0.01

Means ± SEM; * $p < 0.05$ and ** $p < 0.001$ healthy controls versus HD patients (from ref. 17).

It is not conceivable that TML, the first precursor in the biosynthetic sequel of carnitine is limiting, since its extracellular concentration prior to dialysis is considerably higher than that of healthy volunteers[13] (Figure 1). This augmented TML values in uremia might be due to an enhanced release from muscle structure proteins, own to the claimed "dialysis induced hypercatabolism".

A distorted pattern of the plasma carnitine fractions is a common finding in hemodialysis patients[14-17]. Immediately before hemodialysis, highly increased short chain acyl-carnitine concentrations are accompanied with almost normal total carnitine levels and only slightly reduced free and long-chain acylcarnitine concentrations. Thus, the ratio of acylcarnitines to free carnitine is markedly elevated (Table 1).

Possible causes for the increase in the ratio between plasma SCC and FC in hemodialyzed patients are: a) persistent abnormalities of acetyl-CoA oxidation, b) an increased fatty acid availability resulting from acetate and heparin administration during hemodialysis with increased acylation and tissue uptake of free carnitine, c) an enhanced but incomplete mitochondrial oxidation of fatty acids or an increased peroxisomal oxidation of long-chain fatty acids yielding short-chain intermediates[18,19]. Loss of preferential renal excretion of short-chain acylcarnitines and thus accumulation of carnitine esters during dialysis free intervall is not likely resulting in an elevated AC/FC since dialysis induced losses of carnitine are very similar to those seen in the urine from normals.

The chief body store of carnitine is the muscle tissue[12]. Thus, an obvious question is whether the low free carnitine concentrations in plasma are accompanied with a tissue deficit of this substance. Initial investigations repeatedly claimed decreased muscle carnitine stores in HD patients[11,22,23,24]. More recent studies, in contrast, showed normal carnitine concentration in skeletal muscle in this patient category[16,25,26,27] (Table 2). The discrepancies might be due to age and sex differences as well as own to variations in hemodialysis techniques, dialytic age, dietary habits, and, indeed, in the methods of carnitine measurements applied.

Normal muscle values exclude the existence of a secondary muscle carnitine deficiency in these patients. Nevertheless, in some patients very low total carnitine concentrations are observed, especially in patients being treated for many years. This emphasizes the previous claim that carnitine deficiency might be related to the duration of the treatment[28].

THERAPEUTICAL USE OF CARNITINE-SUPPLEMENTATION IN HEMODIALYSIS PATIENTS

Hypertriglyceridemia (type IV hyperlipoproteinemia) has been observed in many patients with chronic uremia[29]. Consequently, many studies are directed to evaluate the clinical

TABLE 2

Muscle total, free and esterified carnitine levels in hemodialys: patients compared to controls.

Carnitine fraction μmol/g NCP	Hemodialysis patiens n = 18	Controls n = 15
Total carnitine (TC)	25.7 ± 8.0	28.8 ± 3.8
Free carnitine (FC)	21.5 ± 7.7	25.2 ± 3.6
Short-chain acyl-carnitine (SCC)	4.10 ± 2.19	3.40 ± 1.85
Long-chain acyl-carnitine (LCC)	0.19 ± 0.19	0.25 ± 0.04
Ratio of AC/FC	0.23 ± 0.17	0.15 ± 0.09

Means ± SD ; NCP = non-collagen protein (from ref. 27).

consequences of a reduced transport of activated fatty acids across the mitochondrial membrane in the face of a possible carnitine deficiency. Further approaches of carnitine deficiency were related to muscle weakness, postdialysis asthenia, muscle cramps, unspecific myopathy, intradialysis hypotension, and a higher incidence of arrhythmia during HD[23].

The currently employed L-carnitine supplementation refers to doses of 15-100 mg/kg body weight. Such a supplementation administered intravenously, orally or via the dialyzate is highly effective in increasing plasma carnitine concentrations. In addition, it is expected that carnitine supplementation should stimulate the oxidation of long-chain fatty acids and thus decrease their availability for esterification to triglycerides[31]. The reported effects of L-carnitine supplementation on lipid metabolism are, however, contradictory. In some studies a lowering of elevated triglycerides and an increase of HDL-cholesterol are described[32,33] while in other studies these effects are not confirmed and occasionally an increase in triglycerides is reported[34,35]. A group of responders and nonresponders was emphasized by Vacha et al.[32]. Patients with hypertriglyceridemia, low levels of high-density lipoprotein-cholesterol and apoprotein A at the lower limit of normal range are rendered as responders whereas those exhibiting hypertriglyceridemia and normal high-density lipoprotein-cholesterol and apoprotein A values belong to the category of nonresponders. Importantly, addition of L-carnitine to the dialysis fluid, presumably the most physiological modus of carnitine supplementation, did not influence hyperlipidemia in HD patients[36].

In recent years a growing body of experimental and clinical evidence indicated that the effects of carnitine are dose-dependent[15,37]. It is suggested that a moderate increase in free carnitine concentration results in a ketogenic effect which in its turn may stimulate beta-oxidation. On the other hand, high free carnitine levels due to excessive amounts given may affect the carnitine carrier system. Actually, an inversion of the key enzymes by the substrate surplus readily induces the formation of intramitochondrial acylcarnitines[21]. These esters might be shuttled from the mitochondria and the peroxisomes via inversion of the carnitine-acyltransferase to the cytosol where fatty acid synthesis takes place, followed by liver triglyceride- and VLDL-synthesis and subsequent accumulation[38].

In consonance with these observations long-term intravenous supplementation with low-dose L-carnitine (5 mg/kg body weight) was investigated in hemodialyzed children with hyperlipoproteinemia of type IV[39]. Carnitine was given at completion of each hemodialysis treatment (3 times a week) over 5 months. Total plasma carnitine concentration raised compared to that before therapy (117.7 ± 33.0 µM vs. 37.9 ± 15.8 µM; $p \leq 0.05$), the free fraction being the chief portion of the difference. Prior to therapy the patients revealed high plasma triglyceride concentrations which were markedly reduced after 5 months carnitine therapy (3.82 ± 1.6 mM vs. 1.86 ± 0.7 mM; $p \leq 0.05$). The initially low HDL-cholesterol levels were increased after supplementation

(0.91 ± 0.2 mM vs. 1.13 ± 0.2 mM; $p \leq 0.05$). Keeping in mind that free carnitine, acylated carnitine, free CoA and acylated CoA are in a dynamic equilibrium, an excessive increase in free carnitine thus can reduce accumulation of acyl-CoA what is indicated by the relatively less increase in the concentration of the acylated fraction (decreased ratio of AC/FC). If the concentration of carnitine and thereby its availability for acylation increases, a large portion of acylgroups can be transfered to carnitine and, thus, regenerate free CoA facilitating a normal oxidative flux[8]. In addition, a diminished amount of acyl-CoA might be beneficial considering the known inhibitory effect of this substance on certain enzymes. The long-term low-dose L-carnitine-supplementation obviously improves the disturbed lipid-metabolism, suggesting an important role of carnitine in uremic children, thus justifying carnitine-supplementation.

CONCLUSION

The inconsistency in treating hypertriglyceridemia in uremic patients by L-carnitine could partly be explained by the different diagnosis and severity of the disease in the patients, variable dosages of carnitine and different duration of supplementation. As L-carnitine is well tolerated, and no major side effects are reported, supplementation can be recommended. Since supplementation with doses between 15 and 100 mg/kg body weight increases plasma and tissue levels impressively, markedly lower doses (1-5 mg/kg b. w.) should be applied. "Low-dose" carnitine supplementation is favoured in treating hypertriglyceridemia to detect ketogenic or antiketogenic effects which probably depend on body carnitine stores and metabolic state of the individual.

In recent studies it was postulated that enhanced provision of the substrate carnitine may force the reaction of the CPT 1 towards the formation of acylcarnitine. Thus, instead of glucose, oxidation of fatty acids can be maintained, resulting in a preservation of the glycogen stores[40,41]. Interestingly, this effect of supplementary carnitine on fat oxidation was apparent both in normal subjects obviously not carnitine deficient and in patients with postoperative carnitine deficiency.

REFERENCES

1. Rebouche, C.J.: Sites and regulation of carnitine biosynthesis in mammals. Fed. Proc. 41:2848 (1982).
2. Frenkel, R.A., and McGarry, J.D.: Carnitine biosynthesis, metabolism, and function. Academic Press, New York (1980).
3. Bremer, J.: Carnitine-metabolism and functions. Physiol. Rev. 63:1420 (1983).
4. Paik, W.K., Kim, S.: Protein methylation: chemical, enzymological, and biological significance. Advanc. Enzymol. 42:227 (1975).
5. LaBadie, J., Dunn, W.A., and Aronson, N.N.: Hepatic synthesis of carnitine from protein-bound trimethyl-lysine. Lysosomal digestion of methyl-lysine-labeled

asialo-fetuin. <u>Biochem.</u> <u>J.</u> 160:85 (1976).

6. Fritz, J.B.: Carnitine and its role in fatty acid metabolism. <u>Adv.</u> <u>Lipid</u> <u>Res.</u> 1:285 (1963).

7. McGarry, J.D.: New perspectives in the regulation of ketogenesis. <u>Diabetes</u> 28:517 (1979).

8. Borum, P.R.: Carnitine function. <u>In:</u> "Clinical Aspects of Human Carnitine Deficiency", Borum, P.R., ed., Pergamon Press, New York (1986).

9. Guarnieri, G., Toigo, G., Crapesi, L., Situlin, R., Del Bianco, M.A., Corsi, M., LoGreco, P., Paviotti, G., Mioni, G., and Campanacci, L.: Carnitine metabolism in chronic renal failure. <u>Kidney</u> <u>Int.</u> 32 (suppl. 22):116 (1987).

10. Bieber, L.L., and Lysiak, W.: Characteristics and functions of short-chain and medium-chain carnitine acyltransferases. <u>In:</u> "Clinical Aspects of Human Carnitine Deficiency", Borum, P.R., ed., Pergamon Press, New York (1986).

11. Böhmer, T., Bergrem, H., and Eiklid, K.: Carnitine deficiency induced during intermittend haemodialysis for renal failure. <u>Lancet</u> i:126 (1978).

12. Corsi, M.: Secondary carnitine deficiency in renal dialysis. <u>In:</u> "Clinical Aspects of Human Carnitine Deficiency", Borum, P.R., ed., Plenum Press, New York (1986).

13. Kohse, K.P., Graser, T.A., Rössle, C., Franz, H.E., and Fürst, P.: Effect of hemodialysis on plasma-free trimethyllysine. <u>In:</u> "Immune and Metabolic Aspects of Therapeutic Blood Purification Systems". Proc. Int. Symp. Trondheim, Karger Basel (1986).

14. Penn, D., and Schmidt-Sommerfeld, E.: Carnitine and carnitine esters in plasma and adipose tissue of chronic uremic patients undergoing hemodialysis. <u>Metabolism</u> 32:806 (1983).

15. Wanner, C., Förstner-Wanner, S., Schaeffer, G., Schollmeyer, P., and Hörl, W.H.: Serum-free carnitine, carnitine esters and lipids in patients on peritoneal and hemodialysis. <u>Am.</u> <u>J.</u> <u>Nephrol.</u> 6:206 (1986).

16. Rössle, C., Kohse, K.P., Kapp, W., Franz, H.E., Glöggler, A., Bergström, J., and Fürst, P.: Disturbed carnitine metabolism in hemodialysis patients. <u>Clin.</u> <u>Nutr.</u> 5 (suppl.1):136 (1986).

17. Wanner, C., Förstner-Wanner, S., Rössle, C., Kohse, K.P., Fürst, P., Schollmeyer, P., and Hörl, W.H.: Carnitine metabolism in patients with chronic renal failure: effects of L-carnitine supplementation. <u>Kidney</u> <u>Int.</u> 32 (suppl. 22):132 (1987).

18. Guarnieri, G.F., Carretta, R., Toigo, G., and Campanacci, L.: Acetate intolerance in chronic uremic patients. <u>Nephron</u> 24:212 (1979).

19. Ricanati, E.S., Tserng, K.Y., and Hoppel, C.L.: Abnormal fatty acid utilization during prolonged fasting in chronic uremia. <u>Kidney</u> <u>Int.</u> 32 (suppl. 22):145 (1987).

20. Vinay, P., Cardoso, M., Tejedor, A., Prud'homme, M., Levelille, M., Vinet, B., Courteau, M., Gongoux, A., Rengel, M., Capierre, L., and Piette, Y.: Acetate metabolism during hemodialysis: metabolic considerations. <u>Am.</u> <u>J.</u> <u>Nephrol.</u> 7:337 (1987).

21. Engel, A.G., and Rebouche, C.J.: Carnitine metabolism

and inborn errors. J. Inher. Metab. Dis. 7 (suppl.
1):38 (1984).

22. Bertoli, M., Battistella, P.A., Vergani, L., Naso, A.,
Gasparotto, M.L., Romagnoli, G.F., and Angelini, C.:
Carnitine deficiency induced during hemodialysis and
hyperlipidemia: effect of replacement therapy. Am. J.
Clin. Nutr. 34:1496 (1981).

23. Salvica, V., Bellinghieri, G., DiStefano, C., Corvaja,
E., Consolo, F., Corsi, M., Maccari, F., Spagnoli,
L.G., Villaschi, S., and Palmieri, G.: Plasma and
muscle carnitine levels in hemodialysis patients with
morphological-ultrastructural examination of muscle
samples. Nephron 35:232 (1983).

24. Moorthy, A.V., Rosenblum, M., Rajaram, R., and Shug,
A.L.: A comparison of plasma and muscle carnitine
levels in patients on peritoneal or hemodialysis for
chronic renal failure. Am. J. Nephrol. 3:205 (1983).

25. Mingardi, G., Bizzi, A., Cini, M., Licine, R., Mecca,
G., and Garattini, S.: Carnitine balance in hemodialyzed patients. Clin. Nephrol. 13:269 (1980).

26. Fagher, B., Cederblad, G., Monti, M., Osson, L.,
Rasmussen, B., and Thysell, H.: Carnitine and left
ventricular function in hemodialysis patients. Scand.
J. Clin. Lab. Invest. 45:193 (1985).

27. Rössle, C.: Untersuchungen zur Physiologie und Patho-
physiologie des Carnitin-Stoffwechsels. Einsatz einer
optimierten radiochemisch-enzymatischen Methode zur
Carnitinbestimmung. Thesis, University of Hohenheim
(1988).

28. Bazzi, C., DiDonato, S., Castaglione, A., Bazzi, C.,
DiDonato, S., Castaglione, A., Corsi, M., and D'Amico,
G.: Carnitine metabolism in short- and long-term
maintenance hemodialysis. In: Clinical Aspects of Human
Carnitine Deficiency, Borum, P.R., ed., Pergamon Press,
New York (1986).

29. Chan, M.K., Varghese, Z., and Moorhead, J.F.: Lipid abnormalities in uremia, dialysis and transplantation.
Kidney Int. 19:625 (1981).

30. Wanner, C., and Hörl, W.H.: Carnitine abnormalities in
patients with renal insufficiency. Pathophysiological
and therapeutical aspects. Nephron 50:89 (1988).

31. Gerondaes, P., Alberti, K., and Agius, L.: Fatty acid
metabolism in hepatocytes cultured with hypolipidaemic
drugs. Biochem. J. 253:161 (1988).

32. Vacha, G.M., Giorcelli, G., Siliprandi, N., and Corsi,
M.: Favourable effects of L-carnitine treatment on
hypertriglyceridemia in hemodialysis patients: decisive
role of low levels of high-density lipoprotein-
cholesterol . Am. J. Clin. Nutr. 38:532 (1983).

33. Zilleruelo, G., Novak, M., Freundlich, M., Goldberg,
R., Abitol, C., and Strauss, J.: L-carnitine supplementation ameliorates hyperlipidemia in children on
hemodialysis. In: "Clinical Aspects of Human Carnitine
Deficiency", Borum, P.R., ed., Pergamon Press, New York
(1986).

34. Nilsson-Ehle, P., Cederblad, G., Fagher, B., Monti, M.,
and Thysell, H.: Plasma lipoproteins, liver function
and glucose metabolism in hemodialysis patients: lack
of effect of L-carnitine supplementation. Scand. J.
Clin. Lab. Invest. 45:179 (1985).

35. Ahmad, S., Golper, T., Hirschberg, R., Kopple, J., Katz, L., Kurtin, P., Ashbrook, D., and Wolfson, M.: Efficacy of L-carnitine in hemodialysis: a multi-center controlled clinical trial. Kidney Int. 31:226 (1987).

36. Yderstraede, K.B., Pedersen, F.B., Dragsholt, C., Trostmann, A., Laier, E., and Larsen, H.F.: The effect of L-carnitine on lipid-metabolism in patients on chronic hemodialysis. Nephrol. Dial. Transplant 1:238 (1987).

37. Böhles, H.J., and Akcetin, Z.: Ketogenic effects of low and high levels of carnitine during total parenteral nutrition in the rat. Am. J. Clin. Nutr. 46:47 (1987).

38. Guarnieri, G., Toigo, G., Situlin, R., DelBianco, M.A., Corsi, M., LoGreco, P., Paviotti, G., Mioni, G., and Campanacci, L.: Carnitine metabolism in chronic renal failure. Kidney Int. 32 (suppl. 22):116 (1987).

39. Glöggler, A., Bulla, M., and Fürst, P.: The effect of low-dose supplementation of L-carnitine on lipid metabolism in hemodialyzed children. Kidney Int. in press (1989).

40. D'Attellis, N.P., Kulapongse, S., Richelle, M., Dahlan, W., Elwyn, D.H., Rössle, C., Fürst, P., and Carpentier, Y.: Metabolic utilization of energy substrates during intravenous L-carnitine supplementation in normal man. Metabolism in press (1989).

41. Sandstedt, S., Cederblad, G., Cennmarken, C., Lindholm, M., Larsson, J.: The effect of L-carnitine supplemented TPN on lipid- and nitrogen-metabolism in critically ill patients. Clin. Nutr. 6 (spec. suppl.):24 (1987).

PATHOPHYSIOLOGY AND TREATMENT OF HYPERTENSION IN DIALYSIS PATIENTS

August Heidland, Roland M. Schaefer

Department of Internal Medicine, Division of Nephrology, Univ. of Würzburg, FRG

PREVALENCE

Before the start of regular dialysis treatment (RDT) the prevalence of hypertension averages between 75 and 90%[1,2]. During long-term RDT its prevalence declines markedly. The resulting inverse relationship between duration of RDT and elevated blood pressure (BP) is not only caused by the early death of hypertensive patients, but mainly due to the antihypertensive effect of dialysis itself. This BP-lowering effect relates only to hypertensive but not normotensive patients. In a 10-year follow-up study the percentage of hypertensive patients declined from 73 to 16 %[3]. Hypertension disappeared in younger individuals, while it persisted or developed de-novo in older patients, showing the characteristics of systolic hypertension. This observation underlines the role of age-related factors in the pathogenesis of this type of hypertension. Interestingly, the prevalence of hypertension after 10 years of dialysis was lower than the prevalence in an age- and sex-matched population [4]. In these patients, besides fluid and salt removal by dialysis, a decrease in the dry weight, observed in many patients after 5 years of dialysis treatment, may contribute to the BP-lowering effect. It appears that **prolonged dialysis sessions up to 24 to 30 hours** per week lead to a more effective control of blood pressure. In a 10-year follow-up study on 52 patients performed by Charra[5] normotension was achieved by strict maintenance of dry weight alone (low salt diet, but no antihypertensive drugs).

During the last several years the percentage of hypertensive patients in RDT-programs seems to be rising. Several factors have been implicated, such as shortening of dialysis time[6], high dietary sodium intake in non-compliant patients, and the use of high sodium concentrations in the dialysate[7]. In a recent multicenter study on 655 patients with a mean time in dialysis of 45 months, 54 % of the patients received antihypertensive drugs[8]. In the future a further rise in the prevalence of hypertension has to be expected due to the widespread use of erythropoietin for the treatment of renal anemia, which has been shown to increase BP in a certain number of RDT-patients.

HETEROGENEITY OF HIGH BLOOD PRESSURE PROFILES IN RDT-PATIENTS

Due to continuous monitoring of blood pressure it has been feasible to identify different groups of hypertensive patients on RDT-treatment. In the majority of patients fluid removal during dialysis (and a fall of plasma osmolarity) cause a decline of arterial blood pressure (volume-dependent hypertension). However, there are patients who show an unchanged BP or even a paradoxical rise due to various pressure mechanisms. After completion of dialysis a progressive decline both in systolic and in diastolic BP with a nadir at 5 hours after dialysis has been reported[9]. Interestingly, the nocturnal decline of BP, observed in healthy subjects and patients with essential hypertension is abolished in many hypertensive RDT patients[10]. This might be caused by an autonomic neuropathy and/or volume expansion.

HYPERTENSION AS A RISK FACTOR OF CARDIOVASCULAR DISEASE

Hypertension is the most important risk factor for cardiovascular disease and atherosclerosis in RDT patients. It contributes significantly to accelerated atherosclerosis, as demonstrated by Vincenti[11] who obtained vascular tissue during transplant surgery in 50 RDT-patients. Capillary morphology is markedly altered in these patients. Using intravital microscopy hypertensive dialysis patients show a significant decreased capillary density and increased percentage of tortuous capillary loops as compared to normotensive patients[12].

In the Diaphan Collaborative Study[13] a survival analysis was performed in 1453 patients on RDT. Elevated blood pressure, in particular diastolic BP, besides age and male sex were significant risk factors for cardiovascular mortality. The relationship between diastolic BP and cerebrovascular accidents was particular obvious. The number of strokes was 1.5 times higher than myocardial infarctions. Surprisingly, body mass index, high cholesterol and high triglyceride levels were not found to be associated with increased cardiovascular mortality. On the contrary, low body mass index, low cholesterol and low urea concentration were associated with increased cardiovascular mortality. In another study on 320 RDT-patients at risk for ischemic heart disease diastolic hypertension and age contributed significantly to its development[14].

MECHANISMS OF HYPERTENSION IN DIALYSIS PATIENTS

Traditionally volume overload and activation of the renin angiotensin system were assumed to be the most important pathomechanisms in hypertension of end-stage renal failure[15]. More recently the contributory role of other factors such as the adrenergic nervous system, hypercalcemia and therapy with recombinant erythropoietin have been implicated.

VOLUME STATUS

The central role of salt and water retention has been underscored by numerous clinical observations. Thus, hypertension can be normalized in about 70 to 80 % by strictly controlling the dry weight[1].

The pathogenesis of the volume-induced hypertension is not totally clarified. First of all, according to the concept of Guyton[16], expansion of intravascular volume will cause elevation of cardiac index, while peripheral resistance is decreased or unchanged. In a later phase, enhanced cardiac output may decline associated with an increase in total peripheral resistance. An alternative explanation is proposed by Blaustein's hypothesis[19] postulating the presence of an oubain-like inhibitor of vascular smooth muscle Na^+-K^+-ATPase, which would result in enhanced intracellular sodium and calcium concentration. This hypothesis is underscored by the finding of digoxin-like activity in the plasma of a great number of patients with end-stage renal disease[18]. In addition a circulating sodium transport inhibitor has been described in essential hypertension[19].

RENIN-ANGIOTENSIN-SYSTEM

Studies of Schalekamp[20], Klaus[21] and Weidmann[22] have indicated that uremic patients with hypertension have abnormally high concentrations of renin and angiotensin II in relation to exchangeable sodium. In patients with refractory hypertension even normal levels of renin and angiotensin II in the presence of sodium excess and increased blood volume are clearly inappropriate. In some patients blood pressure remains high despite the fact that dry weight has been reached by dialysis. In these individuals BP may rise further during dialysis in response to sodium and volume depletion. Thus, hypovolemic hypertension will develop during hemodialysis.

In these patients bilateral nephrectomy has been performed to normalize high blood pressure in the early seventieth[1]. However, this kind of treatment, which may improve blood pressure drastically, leads to a variety of problems with respect to volume homeostasis, blood pressure and erythrogenesis. Due to the availability of a host of powerful antihypertensive drugs, the need for bilateral nephrectomy has been eliminated.

The BP lowering effect of nephrectomy does not prove that the renin angiotensin system is the only cause of hypertension, since in the damaged kidney other hypertensive factors may be generated. For instance, afferent renal nerves could enhance the activity of the sympathical adrenergic system[24]. The most important indication for the role of plasma renin in the pathogenesis of dialysis restant hypertension is shown by Mimran[23] who found a decrease in blood pressure after infusion of the angiotensin II antagonist saralasin, particularly in patients with high initial renin.

ADRENERGIC NERVOUS SYSTEM

In most studies on RDT-patients serum norepinephrine

and epinephrine concentrations are elevated[25-29], while in some other investigations normal levels were reported (Campese[30], Rauh[31], Kettner[32]).

In chronic renal failure numerous factors contribute to alterations of catecholamine metabolism. In rats with experimental uremia synthesis of norepinephrine is decreased due to a lowered activity of tyrosine hydroxylase, while the degradation of norepinephrine in peripheral nerve tissues is enhanced. The neuronal uptake of norepinephrine is reduced, probably due to uremic toxins such as methylguanidine and guanidine[33]. According to these findings, the value of basal plasma norepinephrine levels as an index of sympathetic nervous system activity is limited.

On the other hand, strong evidence has been forwarded for enhanced sympathetic activity as a cause of hypertension in end-stage renal disease:
1. The decline in elevated BP in subtotal nephrectomized rats is much more pronounced after pithing (dissection of medulla oblongata) than in normal rats[34].
2. Blood pressure falls in hypertensive but not normotensive RDT-patients following the administration of the selective sympathetic neurone blocker debrisoquine[35]
3. Mean arterial pressure, heart rate, norepinephrine and epinephrine decrease markedly after administration of clonidine (0,4 mg/d) in hypertensive dialysis patients. Interestingly in these investigations blood volume and plasma renin activity were slightly increased after clonidine administration[36].

Thus, it can be concluded that an enhanced sympathetic tone does contribute considerably to the increased arterial pressure in uremic patients.

As potential causes of the activation of the adrenergic system a stimulation of afferent renal nerves[24] and a reduced baroreceptor activity[37,38]) has been proposed. Furthermore, a reduced central dopaminergic tone has also to be taken into consideration, since the administration of bromocryptine, which stimulates dopaminergic activity, lowers supine BP, norepinephrine and prolactin levels[39]. Thus, dopaminergic control of sympathetic activity may be impaired in RDT patients.

The concept of sympathetic overactivity is further strengthened by the findings of a decreased density of $alpha_2$-adrenoreceptors on platelets and in an reduced responsiveness of $alpha_1$-receptors on vascular smooth muscle[40,41]). As a consequence of stimulated adrenergic system, desensitization or down regulation of adrenoreceptors might occur. In addition diminished vascular response to norepinephrine by an excess of parathyroid hormone has been suggested by Iseki[42] who demonstrated that the reduced pressor response to norepinephrine could be prevented by parathyroidectomy in subtotally nephrectomized rats.

HYPERCALCEMIC HYPERTENSION IN HEMODIALYSIS

Increases in serum calcium have been shown to exert hypertensive effects resulting from a rise in cardiac output and an enhanced total peripheral resistance (Weidmann[43]). Calcium induced hypertension which is particularly pronounced in the presence of renal failure, might be caused by several mechanisms. These include potentiation of the action of vasopressor hormones such as norepinephrine and angiotensin II as well as stimulated catecholamine release at the adrenal medulla and at adrenergic neurons[44,45]). Left ventricular contractility is enhanced[46].

The incidence of hypercalcemic hypertension in dialysis patients is nowadays observed with increasing frequency and might be due to therapy with calcium carbonate and/or vitamin D analogues[47].

PROSTAGLANDINES AND RENOMEDULLARY LIPIDS

Intrarenal prostaglandines are locally active hormones which exert blood pressure modulating effects. PGE_2 and prostacyclin act as vasodilators and influence renin secretion as well as renal adrenergic activity. They are capable of blunting vasoconstrictor stimuli. Thus, their absence may favour a rise in blood pressure.

Moreover, another group of intrarenal substances known as renomedullary lipids may play a certain role in the lowering of blood pressure[48].

ERYTHROPOIETIN TREATMENT OF RENAL ANEMIA

An increase in blood pressure, particular in patients with preexisting hypertension, is one of the consistent adverse effects of erythropoietin therapy of renal anemia[49,50]). In a small number of patients a sudden rise in blood pressure resulted in hypertensive encephalopathy and grand-mal convulsions[51].

The rise in blood pressure probably is not a direct effect of EPO, since there is neither an acute nor any dose-dependent effect of the hormone itself. Apparently, two different factors are involved in EPO-associated hypertension:
1. The enhanced hematocrit levels with a concomitant increase in whole blood viscosity will lead to increased peripheral resistance[52,53])
2. There might be a reversal of the hypoxic vasodilatation due to correction of anemia. In the early seventieth Duling[54,55] described the vasodilating effect of hypoxemia. This situation clearly is abolished after correction of renal anemia which improves peripheral oxygenation markedly[56], thereby facilitating an increase in peripheral resistance.

THERAPY OF HYPERTENSION IN THE DIALYSIS PATIENTS

Even though there are no controlled studies on the beneficial effect of antihypertensive therapy on morbidity and mortality, normalization of elevated blood pressure is one of the main objectives in renal replacement therapy. In this regard it is remarkable that Charra[5] reported on an 85 % survival rate in patients maintained on RDT over a period of 10 years. This was achieved by keeping BP within the normal range.

NON-DRUG TREATMENT OF HYPERTENSION

All major guidelines for blood pressure control in RDT-patients emphasize fluid removal combined with reduced sodium and fluid intake to achieve the "dry weight". To prevent dialysis-induced adverse effects such as hypotensive episodes and muscle cramps, sequential ultrafiltration[57], slow dialysis[5] and bicarbonate dialysis has been recommended. Furthermore, a stepwise decrease in dialysate sodium content to about 136 mmol/l has been claimed. As another approach for removal of excess sodium salt substraction, that means ultrafiltration and infusion of an equal volume of an electrolyte free solution, has been suggested[58].

Impressive improvement in blood pressure control in RDT-patients was achieved by physical exercise[59,60] which was applied even during hemodialysis treatment[61]. Additional advantages of this treatment also results in a rise in maximal working capacity and improvements of hematocrit levels as well as lipid profiles.

ANTIHYPERTENSIVE MEDICATION

If hypertension persists despite strict volume control, antihypertensive drugs have to be administered.

BETA BLOCKING AGENTS

Beta blockers, which reduce the release of renin, appear appropriate in RDT-patients, particularly with renin-dependent hypertension[63]. Some beta blockers such as acebutol, atenolol, nadolol and in particular sotalol cumulate and may thereby cause excessive bradycardia. By contrast, the half-life of propranolol, metoprolol, pindolol and labetalol is unchanged[62].

The beneficial effects of beta blockers on blood pressure are limited by several adverse reactions such as decrease of cardiac output, Raynaud-like symptomes, decreased exercise tolerance and central nervous disturbances. Hypotensive episodes during hemodialysis may occur more frequently due to a blunted reflex tachycardia. Furthermore, beta blocker exert some negative metabolic side effects. After moderate dosis of propranolol, a rise in serum triglyceride levels, particular of the low-density class and a marked decline of high density lipoprotein (HDL) fraction II and III are described[64]. Tissue lipoprotein lipase activity decrease. Even though, erythropoietin production in rabbits exposed to mild hypoxia is reduced by beta blockers[65], no worsening of anemia in RDT-patients was observed (Lindner[63]).

ALPHA₁-ADRENERGIC RECEPTOR BLOCKERS

The most clinical used alpha-blocker prazosin is proved to be effective in controlling hypertension in RDT patients in a dose of about 8 mg/day[66]. Its main hemodynamic effect is the lowering of peripheral vascular resistance while cardiac output is unchanged. It seems that prazosin facilitates beneficial metabolic effects. Thus, triglyceride levels are unchanged, while HDL-3 cholesterol level rise[66].

Tissue lipoprotein lipase activity increases after prazosin. The most important side effect of alpha$_1$-receptor blockers may be postural hypotension in the dialysis patients.

ALPHA$_2$-ADRENERGIC AGONISTS

The central acting sympathicolytic drugs (clonidine, alpha-methyldopa) are highly effective due to lowering the enhanced sympathetic outflow in uremia. Beneficial hemodynamic effects in renal insufficiency have been shown by Levitan[68] and Izzo[27]. Recently, clonidine has also been found to prevent "restless-legs" syndrome in RDT-patients[67].

Since about 50 % of clonidine is eliminated by the normal kidney, its plasma half-life in uremia is prolonged; thus, a dose reduction of clonidine to 50 to 70 % should be performed[62].

The main clinical problem with clonidine therapy is sedation, dryness of the mouth and in some patients brady-cardia and AV-prolongation.

CALCIUM CHANNEL BLOCKERS

Calcium channel blockers are valuable drugs, since their main hemodynamic action is lowering of the enhanced peripheral resistance. They may be of particular value in patients with Raynaud-syndrome which is common in dialysis patients[69]. In own investigations institution of nifedipine therapy resulted in a reduction of systolic and diastolic blood pressure with a maximal effect after 4 weeks of treatment[70, 71]. Similar observations were made after administration of a long-acting verapamil[70, 71]. In both studies a good compatibility was revealed and no tolerance developed.

Fortunately, calcium antagonists exert no negative influence on carbohydrate and lipid metabolism. Cholesterol and triglyceride levels remain unchanged. Surprisingly, administration of nifedipine resulted in a decline of both serum insulin and glucose levels[72] which indicates an improved glucose tolerance. Glucagon and parathyroid hormone levels remained unchanged by the administration of calcium channel blockers. Determinations of Vitamin D metabolites revealed an unchanged 1,25-hydroxy-Vitamin D, while 25-hydrox-Vitamin D showed a significnat rise[73], probably due to stimulation of alpha-hydroxylase activity in the liver cells via reduction of cytosolic calcium.

It appears that the use of calcium antagonists is of particular interest in patients with chronic renal failure in terms of accelerated atherosclerosis in uremia. Thus, in rat experimental studies Baczinski[74] showed that the increased myocardial calcium content induced by parathyroid hormone was abolished by simultaneous administration of verapamil. If similar effects are evoked also in patients with end-stage renal failure, calcium antagonists would become the drug of choice to inhibit cardiovascular calcifications.

ANGIOTENSIN-CONVERTING-ENZYME-INHIBITORS

As early as 1979 the use of ACE-inhibitors in dialysis hypertension was reported by Vaughan et al.[75] and confirmed by Wauters[76] and Röckel and Heidland[77]. Almost all hypertensive patients responded favourably to captopril, even in the presence of normal plasma renin levels.

The incidence and severity of various side effects observed initially nowadays are reduced, since much lower doses are administered.

However, cough, skin-rash, leukopenia and dysgeusia still may be a problem in some patients. A constant finding both after captopril and enalpril is worsening of anemia in chronic hemodialysis patients[79], which improves after discontinutation of ACE-treatment. This type of anemia is not due to enhanced hemolysis, but seems to be related to a decline in erythropoesis, suggested by a reduced number of reticulocytes, which is directly related to the concentration of angiotensin II. Determinations of erythropoietin in plasma showed both unchanged[79] and decreased levels[80].

As angiotensin II has been related to thirst regulation, ACE-inhibitors could exert a potential beneficial action on excessive interdialytic weight gain. In order to investigate this problem two double-blind studies were performed. While one study could not demonstrate any positive effect[81], the other[82] showed that enalapril caused a significant reduction thirst, oral fluid intake and weight gain between dialysis sessions. Thus, more studies are now required to answer the question whether ACE-inhibitors are useful drugs to control interdialytic weight gain.

Since ACE-inhibitors are partly excreted by the kidneys their plasma half life is prolonged in renal insufficiency which requires a dose reduction of about 50 % in the dialysis patients[62].

In summary, due to its negative influence on renal anemia the clinical use of ACE-inhibitors appears to be limited to patients with drug resistant hypertension. Further studies are required to finally evaluate the benefits and risks of this group of antihypertensive drugs.

For treatment of hypertension in dialysis patients calcium channel blockers seem to be the drug of choice followed by beta blockers, central sympathicolytic agents and - in drug resistant hypertension - ACE-inhibitors. In the individual patient the clinical situation (for instance stenocardia) and the profile of side effects will determine the selection of the drug.

REFERENCES

1. Lazarus, J. M., Hampers, C. C. and Merrill, J. P., 1974, Hypertension in chronic renal failure. Treatment with hemodialysis and nephrectomy, Arch. Intern. Med., 133:1050.
2. Weidmann, P. and Maxwell, M. H. 1975, The renin-angiotensin-aldosterone system in terminal renal failure, Kidney Int., 8:219.

3. Degli Esposti, E., Boero, R., Chiarini, C., Nagroni, D., Quarello, F., Santoro, A., Sturani, A., Zuccala, A., Piccoli, G. and Zucchelli, P., 1983, Blood pressure behaviour in hemodialysis patients treated for 10 years, Int. J. Artif. Organs, Vol. 6:121

4. Bellettini, W., Francesconi, F., Bentivogli, M., Cremonini, G., Marchetta, F., Viscanti, G., Autore, A., Bonaiuto, S., Cantadori, L and Piatteli, A., 1976, Contributo allo studio epidemiologico dell'ipertensione arteriosa in provincia di Bologna, Caratteristiche generali, Osp. Vita 6:52

5. Charra, B., Calemard, E., Cuche, M. and Laurent, G., 1983, Control of hypertension and prolonged survival on maintenance hemodialysis, Nephron, 33:96

6. Sellars, L., Robson, V. and Wilkinson, R., 1979, Sodium retention and hypertension with short dialysis, Br. med. J. i:520

7. Levin, N.W. and Grondin, G., 1978, Dialysate sodium concentration, Int. J. artif. Organs, 1:255

8. Langer, K., Raidt, H., Chu, W.T. and Graefe, U., 1988 Drugs prescribed in chronic hemodialysis patients: A multicenter report, EDTA/ERA Congress Madrid, Abstract p. 178

9. Batlle, D.C., von Riotte, A. and Lang, G., 1986, Delayed hypotensive response to dialysis in hypertensive patients with end-stage renal disease, Am. J. Nephrol., 6:14

10. Baumgart, P., Lison, A.E., Gemen, S., Walger, P., Graefe, U. and Rahn, K.H., 1988, Ambulatory 24 h-blood pressure monitoring n renal failure, hemodialysis and after kidney transplantation, EDTA/ERA Congress Madrid, Abstract p. 85

11. Vincenti, F., Amend, W.J., Abele, J., Feduska, N.J. and Salviatierra, O.Jr, 1980, The role of hypertension in hemodialysis associated atherosclerosis, Am. J. Med., 68:363

12. Leunissen, K.M.L., van den Berg, B.W., Noordzij, T.C., Slaaf, D. W. and van Hoof, J. P., 1988, Capillary morphology in chronic hemodialysis patients, EDTA/ERA Congress Madrid, Abstract p. 180

13. Degoulet, P., Legrain, M., Reach, I., Aime, F., Devries, C., Rojas, P. and Jacobs, C., 1982, Mortality risk factors in patients treated by chronic hemodialysis, Nephron, 31:103

14. Rostand, S.G., Kirk, K.A. and Rutsky, E.A., 1982, Relationship of coronary risk factors to hemodialysis-associated ischemic heart disease, Kidney Int., 22:304

15. Vertes, V., Cangiano, J.L., Berman, L.B. and Gould, A., 1969, Hypertension in end-stage renal disease, New. Engl. J. Med., 280:978

16. Guyton, A.C., Coleman, T.G., Young, D.B., Lohmeier, T.E. and DeClue, J.W., 1980, Salt balance and long-term blood pressure control, Ann. Rev. Med., 31: 15

17. Blaustein, M.P., 1977, Sodium ions, calcium ions, blood pressure regulation and hypertension: a reassessment and a hypothesis, Am. J. Physiol., 232:C165

18. Graves, S.W., Brown, B. and Valdes, R., 1983, An endogenous digoxin-like substance in patients with renal impairment, Ann. Intern. Med., 99:604

19. Poston, L., Sewell, R.B., Wilkinson, S.P., Richardson, P.J., Williams, R., Clarkson, E.M., MacGregor, G.A. and De Wardener, H.E., 19881, Evidence for a circulating sodium transport inhibitor in essential hypertension, Br. Med. J., 282 (1): 847

20. Schalekamp, M.A., Beevers, D.G., Briggs, J.D., Brown, J.J., Davies, D.L., Fraser, R., Lebel, M., Lever, A.F., Medina, A., Morton, J.J., Robertson, J.I.S. and Tree, M., 1973, Hypertension in chronic renal failure. An abnormal relation between sodium and the renin-angiotensin system, Am. J. Med., 55: 379

21. Klaus, D., 1976, Pathogenesis of renoparenchymal hypertension, in: Renal Insufficiency, Ed. A. Heidland, H. Hennemann, J. Kult, Georg Thieme Stuttgart, 3

22. Weidmann, P., Beretta-Picolli, C., Steffen, F., Blumberg, A. and Reubi, F.C., 1976, Hypertension in terminal renal failure, Kidney Int., 9:294

23. Mimran, A., Shaldon, S., Barjou, P. and Mion, C., 1978, The effect of an angiotensin antagonist (Saralasin) on arterial pressure and plasma aldosterone in hemodialysis-resistent hypertension patients, Clin. Nephrol., 9:63

24. Katholi, R.E., Wintermits, S.R. and Oparil, S, 1981, Role of the renal nerves in the pathogenesis of one-kidney renal hypertension in the rat, Hypertension, 3:404

25. Brecht, H.M., Ernst, W. and Koch, K.M, 1976, Plasma noradrenaline levels in regular haemodialysis patients, Proc. Eur. Dial. Transplant. Assoc., 12:281

26. Naik, R.B., Mathias, C.J., Wilson, C.A., Reid, J.L. and Warren, D.J, 1981, Cardiovascular and autonomic reflexes in haemodialysis patients, Clin. Sci., 60:165

27. Izzo, J.L. Jr., Izzo, M.S., Sterns, R.H. and Freeman, R.B., 1982, Sympathetic nervous system hyperactivity in maintenance hemodialysis patients, Trans. Am. Soc. Artif. Intern. Organs, 28:604

28. Corneille, L., Lachance, S., Demassieux, S. and Carrier, S, 1983, Turnover of free and conjugated serum catecholamines during hemodialysis, Clin. Invest. Med., 6:11

29. Ratge, D., Augustin, R and Wisser, H., 1983, Catecholamines, renin, aldosterone and arterial pressure in patients on chronic hemodialysis treatment, Int. J. Artif. Organs, 6: 255

30. Campese, V.M., Romoff, M.S., Levitan, D., Lane, K. and Massry, S.G., 1981, Mechanisms of autonomic nervous system dysfunction in uremia, Kidney Int., 20:246

31. Rauh, W., Hund, E., Sohi, G., Rascher, W., Mehls, O. and Schärer, K., 1983, Vasoactive hormones in children with chronic renal failure, Kidney Int., 24:27

32. Kettner, A., Goldberg, A., Hagberg, J., Delmez, J. and Harter, H., 1984, Cardiovascular and metabolic responses to submaximal exercise in hemodialysis patients, Kidney Int., 26:66

33. Hennemann, H., Hevendehl, G., Horler, E. and Heidland, A., 1973, Toxic sympathicopathy in uremia, Proc. Eur. Dial. Transplant. Assoc., 10:166

34. Hennemann, H., 1976, Die urämische Sympathicopathie, Kidney Int., 28:814, Thieme Verlag

35. Schohn, D., Weidmann, P., Jahn, H. and Beretta-Piccoli, C., 1985, Norepinephrine-related mechanism in hypertension accompanying renal failure, Kidney Int., 28:814

36. Izzo, J.L.Jr., Santarosa, R.P., Larrabee, P.S., Smith, R.J. and Kallay, M.C., 1987, Increased plasma norepinephrine and sympathetic nervous activity in essential hypertensive and uremic humans: effects of clonidine, J. Cardiovasc. Pharmacol., 10, Suppl.: 12:225

37. Tomiyama, O., Shigai, T., Ideura, T., Tomita, K., Mito, Y., Shinohara, S. and Takeuchi, J., 1980, Baroreflex sensitivity in renal failure, Clin. Sci., 58:21

38. Heidbreder, E., Schafferhans, K. and Heidland, A., 1985, Disturbances of peripheral and autonomic nervous system in chronic renal failure: Effects of hemodialysis and transplantation, Clin. Nephrol., 22:222

39. Sturani, A., Degli Esposti, E., De March, A., Santoro, A., Fuschini, G., Zuccala, A., Chiarini, C., Glamigni, C. and Zucchelli, P., 1983, Dopaminergic control of sympathetic activity and blood pressure in haemodialysis patients, Proc. Eur. Dial. Transplant. Assoc., 20:156

40. Brodde, O.E. and Daul, A., 1984, Alpha- and beta-adrenoceptor changes in patients on maintenance hemodialysis, Contr. Nephrol., (Karger Basel) 41;99

41. Rascher, W., Schömig, A., Kreye, V.A. and Ritz, E., 1982, Diminished vascular response to noradrenaline in experimental chronic uremia, Kidney Int., 21:20

42. Iseki, K., Massry, S.G. and Campese, V.M., 1985, Evidence for a role of PTH in the reduced pressor response to norepinephrine in chronic renal failure, Kidney Int., 28:11

43. Weidmann, P., Massry, S.G., Coburn, J.W. et al., 1972, Blood pressure effects of acute hypercalcemia: studies in patients with chronic renal failure, Ann. Intern. Med., 76, 741

44. Vlachakis, N.D., Frederics, R., Velasquez, M. et al., 1982 Sympathetic system function and vascular reactivity in hypercalcemic patients, Hypertension, 4:452

45. Boullin, D.J., 1967, The action of extracellular cations on the release of the sympathetic transmitter from peripheral nerves, J. Physiol., 189:85

46. Henrich, W.L., Hunt, J.M. and Nixon, J.V., 1984, Increased calcium and left ventricular contractility during hemodialysis, New Engl. J. Med., 310:19

47. Sica, D.A., Harford, A.M. and Zawada, E.T., 1984, Hypercalcemic hypertension in hemodialysis, Clin. Nephrol., 22: 102

48. Muirhead, E.E., Broos, B., Kosinski, M., Dnaiels, E.G. and Hinman, J.W., 1966, Renomedullary antihypertensive principle in renal hypertension, J. Lab. Clin. Med., 67:778

49. Samtleben, W., Baldamus, C.A., Bommer, J., Fassbinder, W., Nonnast-Daniel, B. and Gurland, H.J., 1988, Blood pressure changes during treatment with recombinant human erythropoietin, Contr. Nephrol., (Karger Basel) 66:114

50. Frei, U., Nonnast-Daniel, B. and Koch, K.M., 1988, Erythropoietin und Hpyertonie, Klin. Wochenschr., 66:914

51. Winearls, C.G., Pippard, M.J., Downing, M.R., Oliver, D.O., Reid, C. and Cotes, M.P., 1986, Effect of human erythropoietin derived from recombinant DNA on the anemia of patients maintained by chronic haemodialysis, Lancet, 11:1175

52. Schaefer, R.M., Leschke, M., Strauer, B.E. and Heidland, A., 1988, Blood rheology and hypertension in hemodialysis patients treated with erythropoietin, Am. J. Nephrol., 8:449

53. Raine, A.E.G., 1988, Hypertension, blood viscosity and cardiovascular morbidity in renal failure: implications of erythropoietin therapy, Lancet, 11:97

54. Duling, B.R. and Berne, R.M., 1970, Longitudinal gradients in periarteriolar oxygen tensin: A possible mechanism for

the participation of oxygen in local regulation of blood
flow, Circulation Res., 27:669

55. Duling, B.R. and Pittman, R.N., 1975, Oxygen tension: De-
    pendent or independent variable in local control of blood
    flow? Fed. Proc., 34:2012
56. Nonnast-Daniel, B., Creutzig, A., Kuhn, K., Bahlmann, J.,
    Reimers, E., Brunkhorst, R., Caspary, L. and Koch, K.M.,
    1988, Effect of treatment with recombinant human erythro-
    poietin on peripheral haemodynamics and oxygenation, Contr.
    Nephrol., 66:185
57. Bergström, J., Asaba, H. and Fürst, P. et al., 1976, Dia-
    lysis, ultrafiltration and blood pressure, Proc. Eur.
    Dial. Transplant. Assoc., 13:293
58. D'Amore, T.F., Wauters, J.P., Waeber, B. and Brunner,
    H.R., 1985, Salt subtraction in patients on maintenance
    hemodialysis. Efficacy and limitations, Am. J. Nephrol., 5:
    275
59. Hagberg, J.M., Goldberg, A.P., Ehsani, A.A., Heath, G.W.,
    Delmez, J.A. and Harter, H.R., 1983, Exercise training
    improves hypertension in hemodialysis patients, Am. J.
    Nephrol., 3:209
60. Goldberg, A-O., Geltman, E.M., Gavin, J.R., Carney, R.M.,
    Hagberg, J.M., Delmez, J.A., Naumovich, A., Oldfield,
    M.H. and Harter, H.R., 1986, Exercise training reduces
    coronary risk and effectively rehabilitates hemodialy-
    sis patients, Nephron, 42:311
61. Painter, P.L., Nelson-Worel, J.N., Hill, M.M., Thronbery,
    D.R., Shelp, W.R., Harrington, A.R. and Weinstein, A.B.,
    1986, Effects of exercise training during hemodialysis,
    Nephron, 43:87
62. Klooker, P., Bommer, J. and Ritz, E., 1985, Treatment
    of hypertension in dialysis patients, Blood Puri., 3:15
63. Lindner, A., Douglas, S.W., Adamson, J.W., 1978, Propra-
    nolol effects in long-term hemodialysis patients with
    renin-dependent hypertension, Ann. Intern. Med., 88:457
64. Meltzer, V.N., Goldberg, A.P., Tindira, C.A., Naumovich,
    A.D. and Harter, H.R., 1984, Effects of prazosin and
    propranolol on blood pressure and plasma lipids in patients
    undergoing chronic hemodialysis, Am. J. Cardiol., 53 (3):
    40A
65. Fink, G.D., Paulo, L.G. and Fisher, J.W., 1975, Effects
    of beta-adrenergic blocking agents on erythropoietin
    production in rabbits exposed to hypoxia, Pharmacol.
    Exp. Ther., 193:176
66. Harter, H.R., Meltzer, V.N., Tindira, C.A., Naumovich,
    A.D. and Goldberg, A.P., 1986, Comparison of the effects of
    prazosin versus propranolol on plasma lipoprotein lipids
    in patients receiving hemodialyis, Am. J. Med., 80:82
67. Ausserwinkler, M. and Schmidt, P., 1989, Erfolgreiche Be-
    handlung des "restless legs"-Syndroms bei chronischer
    Niereninsuffizienz mit Clonidin, Schw. med. Wschr., 119:
    184
68. Levitan, D., Massry, S.G., Romoff, M. and Campese, V.M.,
    1984, Plasma catecholamines and autonomic nervous system
    function in patients with early renal insufficiency and
    hypertension: effect of clonidine, Nephron, 36:24
69. Läppchen, J., Ritz, E., Koch, A., Mörl, H., Bommer, J.
    and Ossenkop, C., Raynaud-Phänomen bei Dialysepatientsn,
    Dt. med. Wschr., 102:521
70. Heidland, A., Riegel, W., Hörl, W., Weipert, J., Geiger,
    H. and Heidbreder, E., 1985, Calcium antagonists: hypo-

tensive and humoral actions in different forms of hypertension, Contrib. Nephrol., (Karger Basel) 49:201

71. Heidland, U., Riegel, W., Heidbreder, E., Hörl, W.H. and Heidland, A., 1986, Calcium antagonists in impaired renal function and hypertension, in: Calcium Antagonsits and Hypertension: Current Status. Ed. J. Rosenthal. Excerpta Medica, Amsterdam, Hong Kong, Princeton, Sydney, Tokyo, 190

72. Riegel, W., Hörl, W.H. and Heidland, A., 1986, Long-term effects of nifedipine on carbohydrate and lipid metabolism in hypertensive hemodialyzed patients, Klin. Wochenschr., 64:1124

73. Riegel, W., Hörl, W.H. and Heidland, A., Long-term effects of nifedipine on plasma levels of 25-hydroxyvitamin D and 1,25 Dihydroxyvitamin D in hypertensive hemodialyzed patients, Klin. Wochenschr., 64:1291

74. Baczynski, R., Massry, S.G. and Kohan, R. et al., 1985, Effect of parathyroid hormone on myocardial energy metabolism in the rat, Kidney Int., 27:718

75. Vaughan, E.D., Carey, R.M., Ayers, C.R. and Peach, M.J., 1979, Hemodialysis-resistant hypertension: Control with an orally active inhibitor for angiotensin-converting enzyme, J. Clin. Endocrinol. Metab., 48:869

76. Wauters, J.P., Waeber, B., Brunner, H.R., Guignard, J.P., Turini, G.A. and Gavras, H., 1981, Uncontrollable hypertension in patients on hemodialysis: long-term treatment with captopril and salt substraction, Clin. Nephrol., 16: 86

77. Röckel, A. and Heidland, A., 1981, Behandlung 'therapieresistenter' Hypertonieformen mit Captopril, Med. Klin., 76:427

78. Sennesael, J. and Verbeelen, D., 1985, Intra-individual comparison of captopril and enalapril in patients undergoing regular haemodialysis, Eur. J. Clin. Pharmacol., 30:257

79. Hirakata, H., Onoyama, K., Hori, K. and Fujishima, M., 1986, Participation of the renin-angiotensin system in the captopril-induced worsening of anemia in chronic hemodialysis patients, Clin. Nephrol., 26:27

80. Kamper, A.L., Nielsen, O.J., Lokkegaard, H. and Strandgaard, S., 1988, Effect of the converting enzyme inhibitor enalapril (E) on hemoglobin (Hb) and plasma erythropoietin (Ep) in patients with chronic renal failure (CRG), EDTA/ERA Congress Madrid, Abstract p. 208

81. Kilpatrick, J.S., DeVault, G., Abreo, K., Brown, S.T., Bairnsfather, L. and Stevens, L., 1988, Effects of enalapril (En) on blood pressure (BP) control and weight changes in hemodialysis (HD) patients, Kidney Int., 13:299 A

82. Oldenburg, B., MacDonald, G.J. and Shelley, S., 1988, Controlled trial of enalapril in patients with chronic fluid overload undergoing dialysis, Br. Med. J., 296:1089

ADJUSTMENT OF DRUG DOSAGE TO HEMODIALYSIS PATIENTS

Frieder Keller, Ulrich Kunzendorf, Holger Hilt*, Anke Schwarz

Freie Universität, Klinikum Steglitz, Abteilung für Allge-
meine Innere Medizin und Nephrologie, Abteilung für Anaes-
thesie und Operative Intensivmedizin, Hindenburgdamm 30
D-1000 Berlin 45, West Germany

PHARMAKOKINETIC PRINCIPLES

Renal failure leads to reduced elimination and prolonged residence in
the body of about one-half of all commonly used drugs. Kidney function
should be taken into consideration for effective but nontoxic drug dosage.
There is no simple parameter to describe kidney function. Glomerular
filtration rate and drug elimination can only be sufficiently evaluated
for clinical purposes by creatinine clearance (CCR). Drug elimination may
be expressed as the rate constant (k) or elimination half-life ($T_{1/2}$ =
ln2/k). The basic law of pharmacokinetics in renal insufficiency says that
all drugs evidence a linear correlation between elimination rate constant
(k) and creatinine clearance (Dettli 1977).

$$k = k_{nr} + a\ CCR$$

The slope (a) and the intercept (k_{nr}) of this equation indicate how
strongly drug elimination depends on kidney function. This linear correlation is also valid for drugs eliminated mainly by tubular secretion
(penicillin) as well as for those subject to extensive tubular reabsorption (lithium).

Drug accumulation after repetitive dosage will be all the greater,
the more elimination depends on kidney function and the more kidney function is impaired. According to accumulation kinetics, a steady state will
be reached after 5 half-lives, when the applied amount is in balance with
the eliminated amount. This steady state is characterized by a maximal
(Cmax), an average (Css), and a minimal (Cmin) concentration. The maximal
concentration is called the peak level (Cmax), the minimal concentration
is the trough level (Cmin). The accumulation kinetics can be calculated
from the dose (D), the volume of distribution (Vd), and the dosage
interval (Tau). The extent of the accumulation depends on the length of
the elimination half-life ($T_{1/2}$).

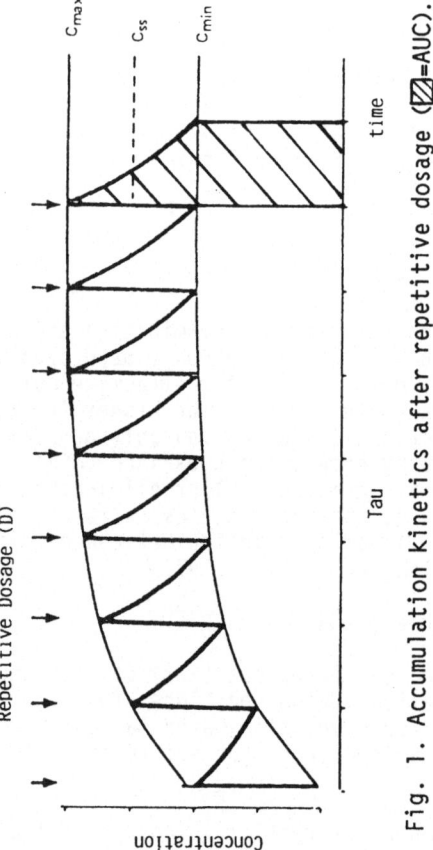

Fig. 1. Accumulation kinetics after repetitive dosage (▨=AUC).

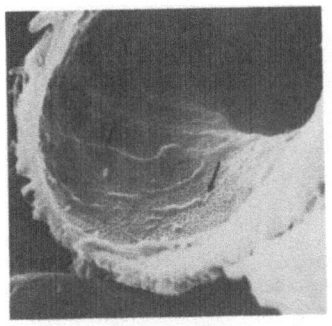

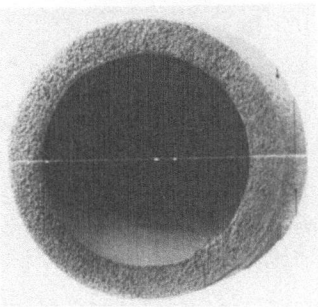

Figure 2. Glomerular capillary simulated by high-flux dialyser capillary.

$$Cmax = \frac{D/Vd}{1 - exp(-0.693\ Tau/T_{1/2})}$$

$$Css = \frac{D/Vd}{0.693\ Tau/T_{1/2}}$$

$$Cmin = \frac{D/Vd}{exp(0.693\ Tau/T_{1/2}) - 1}$$

It is the aim of the adjusted drug dosage to guarantee the normal therapeutic effect. This means that a toxic overdosage and subtherapeutic underdosage must be avoided (Brater 1983). The adjusted drug dosage starts with a loading dose (DL). The loading dose of most antimicrobial agents, for example, corresponds to the normal single dose, since the normal elimination half-life is usually shorter than the dosage interval. Next, the maintenance dose (D) must be reduced according to renal function. The reduced dosage can be adjusted to obtain the same peak concentration (Cmax) or the same area under curve (AUC = Css Tau).

Besides pharmacokinetics, pharmacodynamics must be taken into account. Irreversible acting drugs like aminoglycosides should reach identical peak levels (Cmax) to guarantee the same therapeutic effect (LeBel 1988). Reversible acting drugs like receptor-bound antiarrythmics should aim at an identical area (AUC) to guarantee the normal therapeutic effect. Dose adjustment to the trough levels (Cmin), as suggested in many package insertions of the manufacturers, will lead to subtherapeutic underdosage, since either the maintenance dose will be too small or the dosage interval too long for effective drug action.

If acute or chronic impairment of renal function is advanced to factual or functional anuria, additional elimination must be provided by

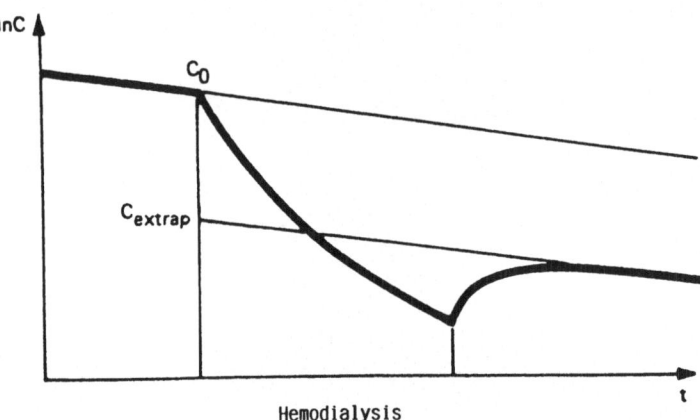

Figure 3. Extrapolation of the eliminated fraction if a rebound occurs after hemodialysis (f = 1 – Cextrap/Co).

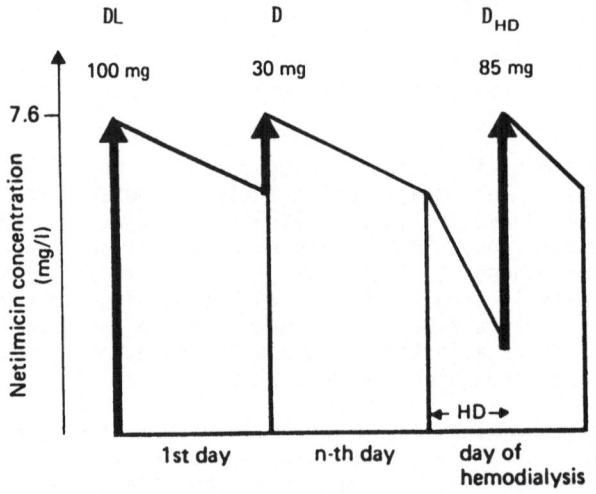

Figure 4. Dosage after hemodialysis (DHD = S + D) consists of the supplementary dose (S = f DL) plus the reduced maintenance Dose (D).

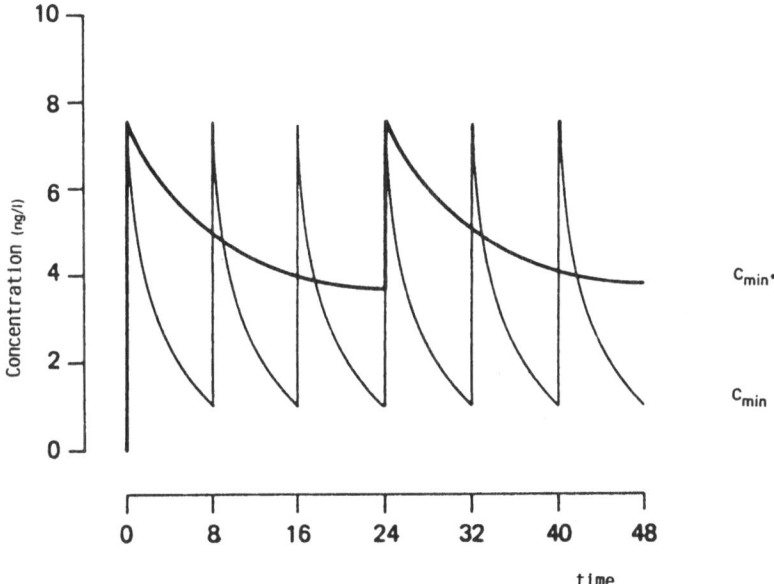

Figure 5. In renal failure, trough levels must be higher than normal.

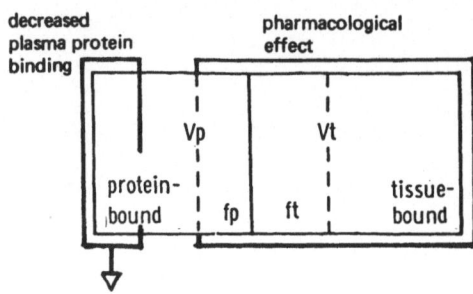

Figure 6. The free plasma concentration remains constant if plasma protein binding decreases.

extracorporeal devices like hemodialysis or hemofiltration. Hemodialysis or hemofiltration capillary filters are conforming more and more to the principles of glomerular capillaries. The pore size of dialysis membranes is 2 to 4 nm and thus corresponds to that of glomerular basement membranes. Hemodialysis comes close to the normal glomerular filtration rate of 130 ml per minute for a period of 4 hours. Drugs eliminated by the kidneys will consequently also be eliminated by hemodialysis.

Hemodialysis involves special problems of drug-dosage adjustment. While necessitating a reduced dosage of renally eliminated drugs, hemodialysis will also readily remove them. The influence which hemodialysis exerts on drug removal of aminoglycosides, some penicillins, cephalosporins, catecholamines and water-soluble drugs is considerable (Gibson 1983). The drug levels required for a therapeutic effect will be lowered to subtherapeutic levels. A supplementary dose (S) of these drugs must therefore be given after hemodialysis.

The effect of hemodialysis on drug elimination can be calculated as the clearance or the removed fraction. For practical dose adjustment, the removed fraction is the superior parameter. The removed fraction is the percentage of a drug eliminated from the body by a standard hemodialysis. Calculation of the eliminative effect is rendered difficult by the rebound phenomenon after hemodialysis. This rebound is due to redistribution from tissue to plasma, since drugs are eliminated from plasma much faster than from tissue stores. The eliminative effect of hemodialysis is overestimated from the decrease in drug levels. Multicompartment kinetics must be assumed. An easier method is to extrapolate the eliminated fraction (f) from drug levels before and after hemodialysis.

To calculate the supplementary dose (S), a standard fixed point is required. The most practical fixed point is the loading dose (DL). Thus, the supplementary dose (S) can be calculated from the loading dose (DL) and the drug fraction removed by hemodialysis (f). This will lead to a slight overestimation of the removed amount corresponding to the non-hemodialyzed fraction of the maintenance dose (D) eliminated before hemodialysis.

The adjustment of drug dosage to hemodialysis patients will be improved by therapeutic drug-level monitoring. Therapeutic drug monitoring should take into account that drug dosage in hemodialysis patients is always a compromise leading to trough levels higher than normal (Rotheram 1988). Trough levels must be higher to guarantee either peak or average steady-state levels identical to those in normal renal function (Cmin* > Cmin). It would otherwise be necessary to prolong the dosage interval and thus also the treatment period. This would be impractical with antimicrobial agents.

Table 1. Netilmicin dosage in normal and anuric kidney function

	normal	anuric
$T_{1/2}$ (hours)	2	48
Vd (liters)	14	14
D/Tau (mg/hr)	100/8	30/24
Cmax (mg/l)	7.6	7.6
Cmin (mg/l)	0.5	5.4
DL = Cmax Vd (mg)	107	107
f		0.50
S = f DL (mg)		55
DHD = S + D (mg)		85

Plasma protein binding and the free plasma fraction of drugs (fp) are the second important aspect of therapeutic drug monitoring in renal failure. Plasma protein binding of those drugs bound to albumin is reduced in renal failure. Decrease of plasma protein binding per se does not require alteration of the drug dosage, since the free plasma concentration (fp C) is unchanged (fp* C* = fp C). The pharmacodynamic effect depends on the free concentration (Bakker-Woudenberg 1985). Alteration of plasma protein binding must, however, be taken into account for therapeutic drug monitoring. In renal failure with reduced plasma protein binding, a lower than normal AUC and a lower trough level should be considered therapeutic (Keller 1987). In renal failure, the effective drug level of phenytoin, for example, is 50 percent lower than normal values.

The pharmacokinetic parameters needed for drug dosage in hemodialysis patients are: 1) the elimination half-life ($T_{1/2}$) to calculate the adequate maintenance-dose (D) reduction, 2) the volume of distribution (Vd) to calculate the desired peak (Cmax) and trough (Cmin) levels, 3) the plasma protein binding and the alteration of the free plasma fraction (fp) to interpret therapeutic drug monitoring, and 4) the fraction eliminated by hemodialysis (f) to calculate the supplementary dose (S). These basic pharmacokinetic data can be found in the literature. We combined them to a tabulated compendium demonstrating that many data are still missing (Keller 1987). Dosage recommendations for hemodialysis patients have been proposed on the basis of such data (Bennett) 1983, Keller 1988). These preliminary recommendations should be improved by computer-aided statistics and clinical studies.

AMINOGLYCOSIDE DOSAGE IN HEMODIALYSIS PATIENTS

We have investigated these dosage recommendations for the amino-glycoside netilmicin. Netilmicin elimination depends entirely on renal function. The elimination half-life ($T_{1/2}$) increases from 2 h in normals to 48 h in patients with anuria. The calculated netilmicin dosage for a hemodialysis patient is a reduced maintenance dose (D) of 0.4 mg per kg body weight. The normal dosing interval (Tau) of 8 h should be prolonged to 24 h. The calculated loading dose (DL) is 1.5 mg per kg. The fraction eliminated by hemodialysis (f) is 50 percent. This effect of hemodialysis should be compensated by a supplementary dose (S) of 0.7 mg per kg. The dosage of 1.2 mg per kg after hemodialysis (DHD) consists of the reduced daily maintenance dose plus the supplementary dose. This dosage aims at the same peak levels as in normals (Cmax), corresponding to a maximal steady-state concentration of 7.6 mg per liter. These peak levels can be achieved only with trough levels (Cmin) of 5 mg per liter but not below 2 mg per liter, as in normals.

Table 2. Adjustment of drug dosage to hemodialysis patients

1) Start with loading dose
2) Reduce maintenance dose
3) Extend dosage interval
4) Same peaks but higher troughs than normal
5) Supplementary dose after hemodialysis

This dosage was given to 50 hemodialysis patients with acute or chronic renal failure (Keller 1986, 1987). They were treated in either the operative or medical intensive care unit or the dialysis and transplantation unit. Mortality was 44 percent and considerably high in this very sick patient group. The main cause of death was uncontrolled sepsis. Nephrologic disease and pulmonary infection were significantly associated with a better prognosis than acute renal failure after major abdominal or vascular surgery. The mean peak and trough levels of the 50 patients were 7.5 mg per liter and 3.5 mg per liter respectively, and thus within the intended therapeutic range. The peak and trough aminoglycoside levels, however, were found to be significantly lower in the 22 non-survivors than in the 28 survivors (Keller 1987).

To examine whether the cause of death was the underlying disease or an inadequate treatment, the success of antimicrobial therapy was evaluated in our study according to clinical criteria, such as fever, leucocytosis, or bacteriologic examination. And again, the peak and trough levels were significantly higher in patients with aminoglycoside treatments judged to be successful than in nonresponders (Keller 1986). However, death and treatment failure could also be explained by differences in the severity of the underlying disease or infection.

To descriminate between these confounding factors, a multivariate analysis was done with the 10 clinical parameters presumed to be the most revelant (Kunzendorf 1988). Univariate analysis revealed 8 significant differences between survivors and nonsurvivors with respect to the severity of the disease and the aminoglycoside dosage. In the multivariate

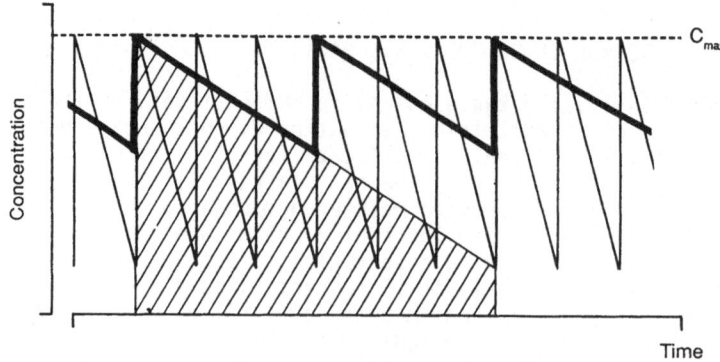

Figure 7. Dosage adjustment to hemodialysis patients (▬) is a compromise between reduced dose, prolonged dosage interval and elevated trough concentrations. Adjustment to identical AUC (▨) will produce a delayed and possibly insufficient effect.

Table 3. Controversial issues of antimicrobial therapy and dosage
adjustment in hemodialysis patients

1) Toxic overdosage versus subtherapeutic underdosage
2) High bolus dose versus frequent intermittent dosage
3) Effective peaks versus toxic troughs
4) Dosage interval and postantibiotic effect
5) Differential increase versus integrated area of concentrations

analysis, 4 parameters were the most important. The need for catecholamines due to severe sepsis and the success of treatment determined
according to infectiologic criteria were two significant discriminators
between survivors and dead patients. The duration of aminoglycoside
therapy and the peak aminoglycoside levels were the two other independent
factors significantly discriminating survivors from non-survivors.

Nephrotoxicity is reversible and of minor importance in hemodialysis
patients. The other risk of aminoglycoside therapy is ototoxicity. Audio-
metry could only be evaluated in 18 patients whose physical condition was
satisfactory. Signs of ototoxicity were found in 3 of them, corresponding
to 17 percent. This incidence is not higher than in patients with normal
renal function (Moore 1984). Aminoglycoside dosage regulation in hemodialysis patients can be considered the most difficult challenge to
pharmacokinetic dose adjustment because of the narrow therapeutic range.
The principles and the clinical results associated with aminoglycosides
could therefore be valid also for many other drugs with a wider therapeutic margin.

In hemodialysis patients, a subtherapeutic underdosage in no less
detrimental than a toxic overdosage. There is an obvious tendency to
underdose aminoglycosides in critically ill patients (Chelluri 1987,
Boettger 1988, Bailie 1988, Franson 1988). Antimicrobial agents should
therefore be given at dosages that achieve the same peak levels as in
normals. The excess of peaks over minimum inhibitory concentration is most
important for effective aminoglycoside dosage (Moore 1987). In hemodialysis patients, these peak levels can be achieved only at the cost of trough
levels much higher than in normals and require that drug therapy be initiated with a loading dose. In addition, the eliminative effect of intermittent hemodialysis must be compensated by applying a supplementary
dosage thereafter.

The maintenance dose should be reduced in renal failure, but not too
much. According to recent aminoglycoside dosage recommendations, the high
single dose is preferable to the low intermittent dosage (Kapusnik 1988,
Wood 1988). The single-dose bolus effect is needed for bactericidal action
(Blaser 1985, Gerber 1986). The dosage interval should be extended to
allow for such a higher single bolus dose. This also makes it possible to
take optimal advantage of the postantibiotic effect lasting for 6 to 8
hours. But the dosage interval should not be prolonged more than
approximately one elimination half-life. For cepha- losporine the
continuous dosage is recommended (Roodendaal 1985, Koenig 1986). But for
the aminoglycosides, the effect most likely depends on the magnitude of
the differential change not on the integrated area. Prolongation of the
dosage interval beyond postantibiotic effect may be detrimental. Aminoglycoside action also depends on the number of peaks achieved.
Anti-infectious therapy is always in competition with time. The delayed
effect could be too late.

REFERENCES

Bailie, G. R., Mathews A., 1988, Quantitative and qualitative assessment of serum concentration monitoring and dosage adjustment of amino-glycosides, <u>Therap. Drug Monitor</u>, 10: 292-295.

Bakker-Woudenberg, I. A. J. M., Van den Berg, F. C., Vree, T. B., Baars, A. M., Michel, M. F., 1985, Relevance of serum protein binding of cefoxitin and cefazolin to their activities against Klebsiella pneumoniae pneumonia in rats, <u>Antimicrob. Agents Chemother.</u>, 28: 654-659.

Bennett, W. M., Aronoff, G. R., Morrison, G., Golper, T. A., Pulliam, J., Wolfson, M., Singer, I., 1983, Drug prescribing in renal failure: Dosing guidelines for adults, <u>Am. J. Kidney Dis.</u>, 3: 155-193.

Blaser, J., Stone, B. B., Groner, M. C., Zinner, S. H., 1985, Impact of netilmicin regimens on the activities of ceftazidime-netilmicin combinations against pseudomas aeruginosa in an in vitro pharma-cokinetic model, <u>Antimicrob. Agents Chemother.</u>, 28: 64-68.

Boettger, H. C., Oellerich, M., Sybrecht, G.W., 1988, Use of aminoglyco-sides in critically ill patients: individualization of dosage using bayesian statistics and pharmocokinetic principles, <u>Therap. Drug Monitor</u>, 10: 280-286.

Brater, D. C., Chennavasin, P., 1983, "Drug use in renal disease,", Adis Press, Sidney, pp. 22-56.

Chelluri, L., Jastremski, M. S., 1987, Inadequacy of standard aminogly-coside loading doses in acutely ill patients. <u>Critical Care Medicine</u>, 15: 1143-1145.

Dettli, L., 1977, Elimination kinetics and dosage adjustment of drugs in patients with kidney disease, <u>Progr. Pharmacol.</u>, 1: 1-34.

Franson, T. R., Quebbeman, E. J., Whipple, J., Thomson, R., Bubrick, J., Rosenberger, S. L., Ausman, R. K., 1988, Prospective comparison of traditional and pharmacokinetic aminoglycoside dosing methods, <u>Critical Care Medicine</u>, 16: 840-843.

Gerber, A. U., Brugger, H. P., Feller, C., Stritzko, T., Stadler, B., 1986, Antibiotic therapy of infections due to pseudomonas aeruginosa in normal and granulocytopenic mice: comparison of murine and human pharmacokinetics, <u>J. Infect. Disease</u>, 153: 90-95.

Gibson, T. P., 1983, Principles of drug dose adjustment during hemodialy-sis, <u>Am. J. Kidney Dis.</u>, 3: 111-113.

Ingerman, M. J., Pitsakis, P. G., Rosenberg, A. F., Levinson, M. E., 1986, The importance of pharmacodynamics in determining the dosing interval in therapy for experimental pseudomonas endocarditis in the rat, <u>J. Infect. Disease</u>, 153: 707-801.

Kapusnik, J. E., Hackbarth, C. J., Chambers, H. F., Carpenter, T., Sande, M. A., 1988, Single, large, daily dosing versus intermittent dosing of tobramycin for treating experimental pseudomonas pneumonia. <u>J. Infect. Disease</u>, 158: 7-12.

Keller, F., Wagner, K., Borner, K., Kemmerich, B., Lode, H., Offermann, G., Distler, A., 1986, Aminoglycoside dosage in hemodialysis patients, J. Clin. Pharmacol., 26: 690-695.

Keller, F., Schwarz, A., 1987, "Pharmakokinetik bei Niereninsuffizienz", Gustav Fischer, Stuttgart, pp. 164-193.

Keller, F., Borner, K., Schwarz, A., Offermann, G., Lode, H., 1987, Therapeutic aminoglycoside monitoring in renal failure patients, Ther. Drug. Monitor, 9: 148-153.

Keller, F., Hilt, H., Haller, H., Walz, G., Kunzendorf, U., Offermann, G., 1988, Arzneimittelverluste bei Hämodialyse und spontaner Hämofiltration, in: Aspekte der Arzneitherapie bei Intensivpatienten, R. Dennhardt, G. Heinemeyer, H. J. Gramm, eds., Springer, Berlin, pp. 55-72.

Koenig, P., Guggenbichler, J. P., Semenitz, E., Foisner, W., 1986, Kill kinetics of bacteria under fluctuating concentrations of various antibiotics, Chemotherapy, 32: 44-58.

Kunzendorf, U., Keller, F., Walz, G., Haller, H., Offermann, G., Borner, K., Lode, H., 1988, Multivariate analysis of aminoglycoside levels in hemodialysis patients, Chemotherapy, 590. (in press)

LeBel, M., Spino, M., 1988, Pulse dosing versus continuous infusion of antibiotics. Pharmacokinetic-pharmacodynamic considerations, Clin. Pharmacokinet., 14: 71-95.

Moore, R. D., Smith, C. R., Lietman, P. S., 1984, Risk factors for the development of auditory toxicity in patients receiving aminoglycosides. J. Infect. Dis., 149: 23-30.

Moore, R. D., Lietman, P. S., Smith, C. R., 1987, Clinical response to aminoglycoside therapy: Importance of the ratio of peak concentration to minimal inhibitory concentration, J. Infect. Dis., 155: 93-99.

Roosendaal, R., Bakker-Woudenberg, I. A. J. M., Van den Berg, J. C., Michel, M. F., 1985, Therapeutic efficacy of continuous intermittent administration of ceftazidime in an experimental Klebsiella pneumoniae pneumonia in rats, J. Infect. Disease, 152: 373-377.

Rotheram, E. B., 1988, Clinical response and peak concentrations of aminoglycosides, J. Infect. Disease, 157: 395-396.

Wood, C. A., Norton, D. R., Kohlhepp, S. J., Kohnen, P. W., Porter, G. A., Houghton, D. C., Brummett, R. E., Bennett, W. M., Gilbert, D. N., 1988, The influence of tobramycin dosage regimens on nephrotoxicity, ototoxicity, and antibacterial efficacy in a rat model of subcutaneous abscess, J. Infect. Disease, 158: 13-22.

PHARMACOKINETIC ASPECTS OF DRUG TRANSPORT IN CONTINUOUS AMBULATORY PERITONEAL DIALYSIS

Norbert Lameire and Severin Ringoir

Renal Division – University Hospital
De Pintelaan 185, B-9000 Ghent, Belgium

INTRODUCTION

Pharmacokinetics involve the study of the time-course of the concentration of a drug or, in some cases, its metabolites, in different parts of the organism. Mathematical models are used to describe this time-course. These models allow prediction of the concentrations as a function of dosage, route of administration and of factors such as disease states. This time-course of the plasma concentrations can usually be adequately described by a model in which the body is viewed as one compartment, in which the drug is distributed rapidly and homogeneously. In a two-compartment model, the body is divided in a central compartment which contains the plasma, but also the extra-cellular fluid of highly perfused organs such as heart, lung, liver and kidney, and a peripheral compartment in which the drug is distributed at the slower rate. Fig. 1 describes the plasma concentration of a drug as a function of time for a one-compartmental and a two-compartmental model, respectively.

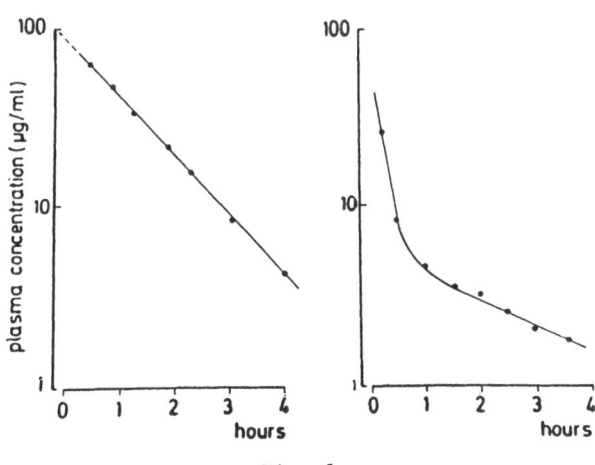

Fig. 1

From the plasma concentrations-time curve, a number of pharmacokinetic parameters can be easily calculated. The elimination half-life of the drug (T $\frac{1}{2}$) is the time needed for the organism to decrease its drug concentration by 50 %.

A closely related parameter is the elimination constant, K_e, where

$$K_e = 0.693 / T \frac{1}{2}.$$

Volume of distribution (V_c) is given by

$$V_c = dose / C_0$$

where C_0 equals the plasma concentration at time of administration. The volume of distribution provides an estimate of the extent of distribution of the drug troughout the body fluid compartments, and of its uptake by different tissues. If there is important uptake of the drug by these tissues, a volume of distribution several times larger than the body fluid volume can be found. The volume of distribution can only be calculated when the dose of the drug entering the body is known, this means when the drug is given intravenously or if the absorbed amount is known exactly.

Total body clearance or plasma clearance is the amount of plasma which is cleared completely of the drug per unit time and gives an estimate of the efficiency of the elimination by organs such as liver or kidney. Total body clearance (Cl) can be calculated by means of the following equation:

$$Cl = 0.693 \times V_c / T \frac{1}{2}.$$

For some substances for which elimination takes place only via the kidney, total body clearance equals renal clearance. Half-life of elimination, in contrast, is dependent not only upon the clearance, but also upon volume of distribution. Although gentamicin and digoxin are both cleared to approximately the same extent as creatinine, this means at a rate of 120 ml/min in a normal situation, half-life of elimination for digoxin is 36 hours, while that of gentamicin is only somewhat more than 2 hours, due to the fact that the volume of distribution of digoxin is more than 500 L, while for gentamicin this is only about 17 L. When elimination in different situation is compared (e.g. patients with renal failure compared to normal, or predialysis patients compared to those on dialysis), plasma clearances should be calculated wherever it is possible. However, intravenous administration of a drug has to be used, except if the amount of absorption is known exactly.

Clearance can also be calculated with the following equation:

$$Cl = D / AUC \text{ where}$$

D is the dose administered and AUC the area under the drug plasma concentration-time curve.
AUC can be determined by the trapezoidale rule.
While pharmacokinetics of a drug are usually studied after

single administration, it is of utmost importance to know
what happens after chronic administration of a drug.
When a drug with a longer half-life is given, an important
fraction of what was introduced with the first administration, will still be present at the moment the second dose is
given. Consequently, the concentration after the second dose
will be higher than that after the first dose and accumulation of the drug occurs. Steady-state concentrations are
only obtained after a number of administrations. The time
to reach steady-state plasma concentrations depends on the
half-life and is approximately four to five times the half-
life of the drug; e.g. for digoxin with its half-life of 1.5
days, this works out at approximately 1 week. If the steady-
state levels are to be achieved earlier, a loading dose has
to be given. The extent of accumulation (i.e. how much
higher steady-state levels will be than the levels after the
first administration), depends on half-life and on dosing
intervals.

PHARMACOKINETIC ALTERATIONS IN PATIENTS WITH CHRONIC RENAL FAILURE

In patients with renal failure, the fate of a drug is
altered profoundly. Most important is the decrease in renal
excretion of a drug; however, it should be kept in mind that
other processes are also affected. Biotransformation of some
drugs can either be decreased or increased in renal failure
patients. There is much interest for alterations in plasma
protein binding of drugs in these patients. For a number of
acidic drugs, which are mainly bound to plasma albumin, binding is often markedly decreased, due to either a decrease
in albumin concentration or to a decrease in affinity at the
binding sites.

These changes will markedly affect the calculated pharmacokinetic parameters. Renal clearance of a drug is usually
decreased in rough proportion to the decrease in creatinine
clearance. If renal excretion is the only elimination route
of the drug, total body clearance will be reduced to the
same extent. For substances which are only partly eliminated
by the kidneys, the alteration in total body clearance will
depend upon the relative importance of renal versus non-
renal elimination. It should, however, not be assumed that
for a drug which is not eliminated via the kidney, total
body clearance is not altered in patients with renal failure; indeed, hepatic clearance can also be affected in
these patients.

In patients with renal failure, the half-life of drugs,
which are excreted wholly or in part by renal excretion, is
inversely related to the decrease in total body clearance.

However, the volume of distribution of drugs in these
patients is often different due to the changes in protein
binding. Therefore, half-life of elimination is not a good
parameter for estimating clearing efficiency. These pharmacokinetic changes will lead to important changes in plasma
concentrations, mainly after chronic administration, if the
dose is not adapted. Concentrations in the body will be much
higher and the time to reach the steady-state will increase.

This explains why in patients with renal failure, a loading dose of several drugs is needed.

PHARMACOKINETIC ALTERATIONS IN PERITONEAL DIALYSIS

For a drug given systemically, plasma and dialysate concentrations can be measured as a function of time. To see how far systemic kinetics are affected by dialysis, volume of distribution, serum half-life and total body clearance (and, in some cases residual renal clearance) can be calculated and compared to the values obtained without dialysis). The amount recovered from the dialysate over a period of time (A_{per}), can be used in assessing the need for dose adaptation. This amount should be viewed in relation to that lost from the body over the same period of time by other routes such as hepatic biotransformation or residual renal excretion. This can be approached by calculating the peritoneal clearance (CL_{per}), from the equation /

$$CL_{per} = A_{per} / AUC\ T1 - T2$$

where A_{per} is the amount recovered in the dialysate over a given time period and AUC_{t1-t2} is the area under the curve over the same time period. The peritoneal clearance should be compared to the total body clearance (Cl). Indeed, the increase in plasma clearance which may occur with dialysis ˙s symbolically represented as

$$Cl = CL_r + CL_{nr} + CL_{per}$$

Where CL_{per} is the peritoneal dialysis clearance of any drug; CL_r is the renal clearance and CL_{nr} is the non-renal clearance. A drug with a low molecular weight (less than 500) and with low plasma protein binding may have a dialysis clearance. However, other characteristics of the drug such as its apparent volume of distribution, the rapidity of its distribution troughout the body and the extent of metabolism or excretion from non-renal sources must be considered. One accepts that the dialysability of a drug, in any dialysis strategy, is only clinically relevant when at least two conditions are fulfilled. First, the dialysis clearance should be at least 50 % higher than the total plasma clearance in end stage renal failure without dialysis; otherwise the additive effect of dialysis clearance on overall drug elimination is trivial. Second, the distribution volume of the drug should be less than 1 liter per Kg body weight. If the apparent volume of distribution is large, (greater than 1 liter per Kg body weight), only a small fraction of the drug is available in the plasma for elimination via dialysis. Many studies on peritoneal pharmacokinetics after systemic administration of a great variety of drugs have been extensively summarized elsewhere (1-3).

Table 1 compares total body clearances and peritoneal clearances of selected drugs after systemic administration in CAPD patients.

TABLE 1. TOTAL BODY CLEARANCES AND PERITONEAL CLEARANCES
OF SELECTED DRUGS AFTER SYSTEMIC
ADMINISTRATION IN CAPD

	Total body clearance ml/min	Peritoneal clearance ml/min	References
Cefamandole	21.9±9.7	0.92±0.25	4
Cefotiam	20.9±3.8	3.3±0.2	5
Cefsulodin	14.7±5.4	4.3±1.7	5
Fosfomycin	7.0±1.4	3.2±0.2	6
Aztreonam	23.8	2.1	7
Cefotaxime	65±25	2.4	8
Vancomycin	9.4±1.9	1.48±0.36	9
Cimetidine	167±20	2.7±0.9	10
Digoxin	28.4	2.74	11

All results indicate negligible low peritoneal clearances compared to plasma clearances after systemic administration of these drugs in CAPD.

Peritoneal clearances of most, if not all drugs, ranged between 0 and 5 ml/min. These results can be explained by a number of factors, determining elimination of drugs during CAPD. The most important is the low dialysate flow rate in CAPD which is around 6 to 7 ml/min. Small solute peritoneal clearances are largely dialysate-flow dependent (12). This explains why rapid exchange peritoneal dialysis, as in IPD, increases low solute clearances. As shown in table 2, the peritoneal clearances of selected drugs are higher in IPD than in CAPD, due to the higher dialysate flow rates.

TABLE 2. PERITONEAL CLEARANCES (ml/min) OF SELECTED
DRUGS IN IPD AND CAPD (13)

	IPD	CAPD
Amikacin	7-15	4-5
Cefamandole	9-12	2-5
Cefotaxime	3-9	2-4
Ceftazidime	5-11	3-4
Cefalexine	12-18	2-3
Gentamicin	10-20	2-3
Metronidazole	13-18	4-6
Tobramycin	10-20	3-5
Vancomycin	5-10	1-3
Cimetidine	3-10	1-3
Quinidine	1-2	0.5-1
Theophylline	10-15	1-2
Digoxin	8-10	3-5

In CAPD , the transport of small solutes per unit of time is small because diffusion equilibrium is either obtained or approached before the dialysate is changed.

**TABLE 3. FACTORS AFFECTING DRUG ELIMINATION AFTER
SYSTEMIC ADMINISTRATION IN CAPD (3)**

<u>Dialysis properties</u>

<u>Dialysate flow rate</u>

Temperature of dialysate
pH of dialysate
Osmotic content of dialysate

<u>Drug properties</u>

Ionic charge
Protein binding
Distribution volume
Extra-renal clearance
Lipid or water solubility

<u>Patient characteristics</u>

Membrane surface
Permeability of membrane
Peritoneal blood flow
Residual renal clearance

Many other factors which play a role in the transperitoneal transport of drugs after systemic administration are
summarized in table 3.

However, by far the result is determined by the low
dialysate flow rate, explaining why peritoneal drug clearances after systemic administration cannot exceed values
higher than 6 to 7 ml/min. Since in terminal chronic renal
failure, the total drug plasma clearance is usually higher
than 20 to 30 ml/min. (table 1) and/or the distribution volume is more than 1 liter/Kg body weight, peritoneal drug
clearance almost never contributes significantly to drug
removal.

Therefore, dose adaptations for CAPD beyond the
recomendations for terminal chronic renal failure are not
necessary. The question then arises whether in the future
peritoneal pharmacokinetic studies in CAPD after systemic
administration of drugs are still worthwile to perform. In
general, for drugs that are pharmacokinetically not influenced by chronic renal failure, CAPD will certainly not
exert a significant influence on their pharmacokinetics.

For drugs that are renally eliminated, a simple determination of their concentration in the drained dialysate in
relation to their plasma level at the same moment should be
sufficient. The low peritoneal drug clearances do, of
course, not exclude the fact that therapeutically effective
concentrations in the dialysate, of for example an antibiotic may be achieved after systemic administration. Due
to the low volume (2 liters) in which the drug diffuses, a
meaningfull concentration can be obtained even with a low
clearance.

The calculated peritoneal clearance after systemic administration is a net clearance and gives an estimate of the net drug transport into the peritoneal cavity. After a dwell time of 5 to 6 hours, an equilibrium between plasma and dialysate is approached and the net clearance gives only the net difference between transfers to and from the body and the two-liter dialysate bag. According to a recently described pharmacokinetic model by Janicke et al. (14) it is possible to evaluate, based on simple mass balance the bidirectional transport processes by calculating time-independent one-way instantenous clearances between the peritoneal cavity and the circulation. These clearances are called distributional clearances. For example, the distributional clearances of Cefamandole (Cl_{D1} and Cl_{D2}) were identical with approximately 16 ml/min., although the net clearance was negligible with only 2 ml/min. In children in IPD, Jusko et al. (15) have reported Cl_{D1} values for gentamicin two- to threefold greater than Cl_{D2} values. In a recent study with Cefotiam and Cefsulodine distributional clearances were 14 ml/min. and 17 ml/min. respectively with net peritoneal clearances of 3.3 and 4.3 ml/min. (5).

This method of calculation is simple, does not require computer-fitting of the model equations and is independent of the number of compartments of the mammelary model used. Data can be derived from analysis during one dwell period only.

INTRAPERITONEAL ADMINISTRATION OF DRUGS

Table 4 summarizes the most important factors that influence the transperitoneal pharmacokinetics of intraperitoneally administered drugs.

TABLE 4. FACTORS AFFECTING TRANSPERITONEAL DRUG
ABSORPTION AFTER IP ADMINISTRATION

DRUG PROPERTIES

Lipid or water solubility
Molecular weight
Charge
Protein binding
Distribution volume
Membrane binding

DIALYSIS PROPERTIES

Dialysate flow rate
Dialysate volume
Temperature of dialysate
Chemical composition of dialysate

PERITONEAL MEMBRANE PROPERTIES

Surface blood flow
Surface area
Peritonitis
Peritoneal sclerosis
Stagnant layers

The low peritoneal clearance of drugs after systemic application is in contrast with the rapid drug invasion out of peritoneum when drug is given via the peritoneal route. This has been explained by assuming an unidirectional transperitoneal drug movement from the peritoneal cavity towards the blood. This is however merily the consequence of two important pharmacokinetic factors. First, there is the large difference between the small dialysate volume and the much larger distribution volume in the body (16,17). This will lead to a high concentration gradient between the two compartments. Second, the sometimes high protein binding of the drug in the plasma versus a negligible protein binding in the dialysate further promotes this apparent one-way diffusion from dialysate to blood. As reviewed by a number of authors, intraperitoneal antibiotics show a systemic absorption varying from 50 to 80 % within a dwell period of 6 hours (1,2). This percentage absorbed after IP administration can easily be obtained by subtracting from the amount of drug initially instilled the total amount of drug that is present in the first peritoneal outflow. Yet, this assumes that there is no decomposition of the drug over the same time interval in the dialysate. A recent study has found that most cephalosporines show a considerable decomposition after 6 hours at 37 °C (18). This may lead to an overestimation of the amount of drug absorbed after IP administration. Besides the composition of a simple drug in dialysate, interaction with other drugs, instilled together merely influences the speed of absorption. For example, simultaneous intraperitoneal administration of heparin and gentamicin, significantly increases the absorption of the latter (19).

The absorption kinetics of a drug given extravascularly is directly proportional with the exchange surface and inversily related to the volume of fluid at the absorption sites (20). This may explain why for example, the absorption of intraperitoneal insulin is greater when injected into the empty peritoneal cavity rather than into the instilled dialysate (21).

Previous studies by us and others have demonstrated a faster and higher absorption of peritoneal drug transfer during peritonitis compared to non-peritonitis for gentamicin, tobramycin and cefuroxim (22-24). This has not been observed with other antibiotics such as cefsulodine (25). Table 5 provides unpublished data on the transperitoneal absorption and the peak plasma levels after intraperitoneal administration of netilmycin during peritonitis and after cure in 6 patients over a dwell time of 6 hours.

As with gentamicin, it can be noted that the percent absorption and the peak plasma levels were higher during peritonitis. For gentamicin, equal concentrations in serum and dialysate were achieved at approximately 24h (22). If a drug, after intraperitoneal instillation is only negligibly cleared after transport to the systemic circulation, as is the case in renal failure for drugs which are mainly excreted via the urine, systemic accumulation of the drug will occur. It has been known that after chronic administration of gentamicin in the dialysate for 2-3 weeks, plasma

TABLE 5. TRANSPERITONEAL ABSORPTION AND PEAK PLASMA
LEVELS AFTER IP NETILMYCIN (500 mg/l)

	Percent absorption (%)	Peak plasma level (ng/ml)
Peritonitis n : 7	83.5 ± 3.4	4.39 ± 0.54
Non-Peritonitis n : 6	67.1 ± 3.1	2.58 ± 0.23

concentrations approach dwell-time dialysate concentrations. This can lead to potentially toxic concentrations and necessitates dose reduction (22). Molecular charge may also influence the transperitoneal absorption. Heparin is a strongly positive electrostatically charged molecule. Because its positive charge prevents absorption, IP heparin rarely affects systemic coagulation (26).

EFFECTS OF DRUG PROTEIN BINDING IN PERITONEAL DIALYSIS

The serum protein binding of drugs may be effected by terminal chronic renal failure. The binding of acidic drugs, which bind almost exclusively to albumin, is usually decreased, due to hypoalbuminemia, the presence of endogenous inhibitors or structural changes of the albumin molecules (27). Unfortunately, few studies exist where the influence of peritoneal dialysis, notably CAPD, on drug protein binding have been assessed. It is generally agreed that changes in drug protein binding during peritoneal dialysis are likely to be secondary to the nutritional status of the patient, as reflected by serum protein concentrations in the low normal range, the resultant peritoneal losses of protein during the dialysis process, and the accumulating endogenous compounds that may be displace highly-bound drugs. The influence of protein binding changes on the total and free concentrations of digitoxin has been reported for CAPD and control hemodialysis patients (28). The protein binding of digitoxin during CAPD was 94.7 ± 1.5 %, significantly less than the 96.2 ± 1.3 % observed binding in control hemodialysis patients. Following a 0.1 mg daily oral dose of digitoxin, the mean free serum concentrations in CAPD and hemodialysis of 0.8 and 0.9 ng/ml, were however not significantly different. It can be expected in general that drugs with a high protein binding usually show a very modest CAPD clearance after systemic administration. When a drug is given intraperitoneally, a higher transport rate will be found, since the concentration gradient is better maintained by the high serum protein binding of the drug.

Most basic drugs mainly bind to alpha 1 - acid glycoprotein (alpha-1-AGP) and in renal failure their binding may be increased, due to the elevated alpha-1-AGP concentrations (29).

A recent study performed in our laboratory has explored the influence of CAPD on the concentrations of alpha-1-AGP

in serum and dialysate and on the serum binding of 2 basic
drugs (oxprenolol and propranolol) and one acid drug phenytoin (30).

Before starting CAPD treatment, the serum binding of
oxprenolol and propranolol was higher and that of phenytoin
lower than in healthy volunteers. This was related to the
elevated serum levels of alpha-1-AGP concentrations in
uremia. During the first week after starting CAPD, the serum
alpha-1-AGP concentrations rose with a concommittent
increase in the binding of oxprenolol and propranolol;
subsequently however, the alpha-1-AGP levels and the binding
of oxprenolol and propranolol decreased to the values found
before starting CAPD. The binding of phenytoin, which was
lower than in normal healthy volunteers, did not show any
change during CAPD. The concentrations of alpha-1-AGP in
dialysate were only two to five percent of that in the
serum. Overall, the changes in protein binding during the
CAPD treatment for the three tested drugs were very small,
around only two percent. For phenytoin the change was from
85 % to 89 %; for the two basic drugs, protein binding in
terminal renal failure, before CAPD, was already more than
93 %, so a further increase of 2 % is not important. In any
case, monitoring total drug concentration might be misleading if the pharmacological or toxic effects of the drug
are due to the free drug concentrations in serum or plasma.

REFERENCES

1. Lameire, N., Bogaert, A.M. and Belpaire, F.M.: Perito-
    neal pharmacokinetics and pharmacological manipulation
    of peritoneal transport. In: Continuous Ambulatory
    Peritoneal Dialysis, Gokal, R., ed., Churchill Living-
    stone, Edinburgh, p. 56 (1986).
2. Paton, T.W., Cornish, W.R., Manuel, M.A., and Hardy,
    B.G.: Drug therapy in patients undergoing peritoneal
    dialysis. Clinical pharmacokinetic considerations.
    Clin. Pharmacokinet. 10:40 (1985).
3. Baumelou, A., Singlas, E., Merdjan, H., Martre, H.,
    Brouard, R., Bentchikou, A. and Rottembourg, J.:
    Pharmacocinétique des médicaments administrés par voie
    générale chez les malades traités par dialyse périto-
    néale continue ambulatoire. In: Séminaires d'Uro-
    Néphrologie, Legrain, M. and Chatelain, C., eds,
    Masson, Paris 11:124 (1985).
4. Bliss, M., Mayersohn, M., Arnold, T., Logan, J.,
    Michael, U.F. and Jones, W.: Disposition kinetics of
    cefamandole during continuous ambulatory peritoneal
    dialysis. Ann. Microbiol. Agents Chemother. 29:649
    (1986).
5. Brouard, R., Tozer, T.N., Merdjan, H., Guillemin, A.,
    and Baumelou, A.: Transperitoneal movement and pharma-
    cokinetics of cefotiam and cefsulodin in patients on
    continuous ambulatory peritoneal dialysis. Clin.
    Nephrol. 30:197 (1988).
6. Bouchet, J.L., Albin, H., Quentin, C.L., de Barbeyrac,
    B., Vinson, G., Martin-Dupont, Ph., Poteaux, L., and
    Aparicio, M.: Pharmacokinetics of intravenous and in-
    traperitoneal fosfomycin in continuous ambulatory peri-
    toneal dialysis. Clin. Nephrol. 29:35 (1988).

7. Bolton, N.D., Gerig, J.S., Scheld, W.M., Swabb, E.A., and Boltou, W.K.: Peritoneal transfer of aztreonam in patients during continuous ambulatory peritoneal dialysis. Kidney Int. 25:255 (1984).

8. Alexander, D., Gambertoglio, J., Barrière, S., Warnock, D., and Schoenfeld, P.: Cefotaxime pharmacokinetics during continuous ambulatory peritoneal dialysis. Clin. Pharmacol. Ther. 35:255 (1984).

9. Bunke, C.M., Aronoff, G.R., Brier, M.E., Sloan, R.S., and Luft, F.C.: Vancomycin kinetics during continuous ambulatory peritoneal dialysis. Clin. Pharmacol. Ther. 34:631 (1983).

10. Paton, T.W., Manuel, M.A., and Walker, S.E.: Cimetidine disposition in patients in continuous ambulatory peritoneal dialysis. Perit. Dial. Bull. 2:73 (1982).

11. De Paepe, M., Belpaire, F., and Bogaerts, Y.: Pharmacokinetics of digoxin in CAPD. Clin. Exp. Dial. Aphereris 6:65 (1982).

12. Rubin, J., Adair, C., and Bower, J.: Dialysate flow rate and peritoneal clearance. Am. J. Kidney Dis. 4:260 (1984).

13. Singlas, E., and Lebelle, A.V.: Extraction des médicaments par la dialyse. Therapie 42:529 (1987).

14. Janicke, D.M., Morse, G.D., Apicella, M.A., Jusko, W.J., and Walshe, J.J.: Pharmacokinetic modeling of bidirectional transfer during peritoneal dialysis. Clin. Pharmacol. Ther. 40:209 (1986).

15. Jusko, W.J., Baliah, T., Kim, K.H., Gerbracht, L.M., and Yaffe, S.J.: Pharmacokinetics of gentamicin during peritoneal dialysis in children. Kidney Int. 9:430 (1976).

16. Rogge, M.C., Johnson, C.A., Zimmerman, S.W., and Wellig, P.G.: Vancomycin disposition during continuous ambulatory peritoneal dialysis: a pharmacokinetic analysis of peritoneal drug transport. Antimicrob. Agents Chemoth. 27:578 (1985).

17. Keller, E.: Peritoneal pharmacokinetics of different drugs. Clin. Nephrol. 30:S24 (1988).

18. Janknegt, R., Koks, C.H.W., and Nube, M.J.: Stability of antibiotics in CAPD fluid. Perit. Dial. Bull. 5:78 (1985).

19. Ponce, S.P., Barata, J.D., and Santos, R.: Interference of heparin with peritoneal solute transport. Nephron 39: 47 (1985).

20. Rowland, M., and Tozer, T.N.: Clinical pharmacokinetics. Concepts and application. Lea and Febiger (1980).

21. Balducci, A., Slama, G., Rottembourg, J., Baumelou, A., and Delage, A.: Intraperitoneal insulin in uraemic diabetics undergoing continuous ambulatory peritoneal dialysis. Brit. Med. J. 283:1021 (1981).

22. De Paepe, M., Lameire, N., Belpaire, F.M., and Bogaert, M.: Peritoneal pharmacokinetics of gentamicin in man. Clin. Nephrol. 19:107 (1983).

23. Rubin, J., Deraps, G.D., Walsh, D., Adair, C., and Bower, J.: Protein losses and tobramycin absorption in peritonitis treated by hourly peritoneal dialysis. Am. J. Kidney Dis. 8:124 (1986).

24. Mc Intosh, M.E., Smith, W.G.J., Junor, B.J.R., Forrest, G., and Brodie, M.J.: Increased peritoneal permeability in patients with peritonitis undergoing continuous am-

bulatory peritoneal dialysis. <u>Eur. J. Clin. Pharmacol.</u>
28:187 (1985).

25. Baumelou, A., Brouard, R., Merdjan, H., Guillemin, A.,
    and Rottembourg, J.: Administration interpéritonéale
    des médicaments au cours de la dialyse péritonéale con-
    tinue ambulatoire. A propos d'une étude cinétique de la
    cefsulodine. <u>In:</u> Séminaires d'Uro-Néphrologie.
    Chatelain, C. and Legrain, M., eds, Masson, Paris,
    12:147 (1986).

26. Furman, K.I., Gomperts, E.D., and Hockley, J.: Activity
    of intraperitoneal heparin during peritoneal dialysis.
    <u>Clin. Nephrol.</u> 9:15 (1978).

27. Tillement, J.P., Houin, G., Zini, R., Urien, S.,
    Albengres, E., Barré, J., Lecomte, M., D'Athis, Ph.,
    and Sebille, B.: The binding of drugs to blood plasma
    macromolecules. Recent advances and therapeutic
    significance. <u>In:</u> Advances in Drug Research, Testa, B.,
    ed., Academic Press, London, p. 59 (1984).

28. Peters, U., Risler, T., and Grabensee, B.: Pharmacoki-
    netics of digoxin with end-stage renal failure treated
    with continuous ambulatory peritoneal dialysis. <u>Kidney
    Int.</u> 20:159 (1981).

29. Haughey, D.B., Kraft, C.J., Matzke, G.R., Keane, W.F.,
    and Halstenson, C.E.: Protein binding of disopyramide
    and elevated alpha-1 acid glycoprotein concentrations
    in serum obtained from dialysis patients and renal
    transplant recipients. <u>Am. J. Nephrol.</u> 5:35 (1985).

30. Belpaire, F.M., Van de Velde, E.J., Fraeyman, N.H.,
    Bogaert, M.G., and Lameire, N.: Influence of continuous
    ambulatory peritoneal dialysis on serum alpha-1 acid
    glycoprotein concentration and drug binding. <u>Eur. J.
    Clin. Pharmacol.</u> 35:339 (1988).

DRUG THERAPY DURING CONTINUOUS ARTERIOVENOUS HEMOFILTRATION

Erich Keller

Department of Medicine , Division of Nephrology
University of Freiburg, FRG

INTRODUCTION

Since the first description of continuous arteriovenous
hemofiltration as a method of emergency fluid removal (Kramer
et al. 1977), this measure has gained wide acceptance predominantly as a supportive treatment of acute renal failure in
critically ill patients. It has been shown that the machine-
free hemofiltration allows liberal parenteral nutrition
without the risk of fluid overload. In addition it has some
capacity to remove uremic toxins. The method can be applied
without sophisticated apparative equipment and without trained
dialysis personal being familiar with the problems of extracorporal circulation.

The technical device consists of a small volume hemofilter connected by an arterial and venous line with two
catheters, placed usually in the femoral vein and artery
(Fig. 1). Blood flow through the filter and filtration across
the capillary wall is driven by the arteriovenous pressure
difference. The blood flow rate through the filter measures
approximately 80 ml/min, allowing 5 to 10 ml ultrafiltrate to
be generated per minute. Anticoagulation is accomplished by
continuous infusion of heparin into the arterial line. Excess
fluid loss is replaced by infusion of an electrolyte solution
into the venous port. As modifications of this method venovenous hemofiltration with a pump forcing the blood through
the extracorporal system and arteriovenous hemodialysis with
dialysate passing the ultrafiltrate compartment have been
described (Stevens et al. 1988).

Drug therapy in critically ill patients is complicated by
(1) the usually unknown pharmacokinetics of drugs in this
particular group of patients suffering from one ore more organ
failures, (2) the possibility of multiple drug interactions
during polypragmatic pharmacologic therapy frequently needed

in these patients, and (3) by the possibility of an altered
relation between the plasma drug concentration and the pharmacodynamic effect (Bodenham et al. 1988). Drug elimination by
continuous arteriovenous hemofiltration may further complicate
the therapeutic situation. Published data on drug elimination
by CAVH are limited to some spare reports (reviews by Golper
et al. 1985 and Hilt and Keller 1987). However, it will be
demonstrated here that it is possible to predict the impact of
continuous hemofiltration on overall drug elimination even in
the absence of proper investigations. This is possible on the
basis of already published pharmacokinetic data of these
selected drugs obtained from patients with renal failure, and
on the basis of some general pharmacokinetic considerations.

CAVH AND DRUG ELIMINATION

The major factors determining drug elimination by CAVH
are: (1) the ultrafiltration rate, (2) the relation of the
drug clearance by CAVH to the total clearance of the drug,
(3) the sieving coefficient or the free filterable portion of
the drug which is not bound to plasma proteins and (4) the
drug`s volume of distribution.

Ultrafiltration Rate and Extracorporal Clearance

The first parameter, the ultrafiltration rate, depends on
multiple factors for example blood pressure, vascular access,
blood flow in the extracorporal system, filter membrane,
hematocrit and others (review by Bozkurt and Hörl 1987). In
continuous arteriovenous hemofiltration the ultrafiltration
rate usually does not exceed 10 ml/min. In our study on the
pharmacokinetics of the fixed combination of Imipenem/
Cilastatin in 10 critically ill patients on CAVH, the mean

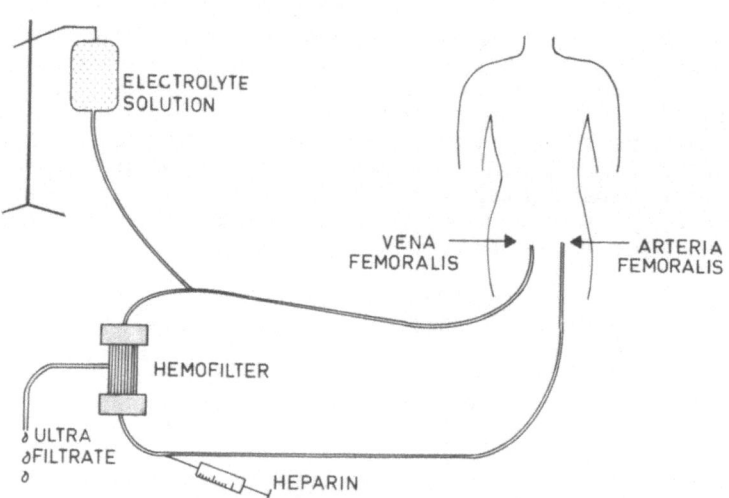

Fig. 1.   Schematic representation of continuous arteriovenous
          hemofiltration (CAVH).

ultrafiltration rate during the sampling time averaged
6 ml/min (Keller et al. 1988). Since active secretion does not
occur in hemofiltration, convective transport is the only
driving force for drug elimination. Thus the extracorporal
clearance of a drug will not exceed this rather low value of
approximately 6 ml/min. If all drug can traverse freely the
membrane, ultrafiltration rate and drug clearance by hemofiltration are identical.

Fraction of the Drug Dose Removed by CAVH

For practical purposes, not the drug clearance but the
fraction of the dose eliminated by CAVH is the most important
information derived from pharmacokinetic studies. With this
information the clinician may calculate the amount of drug
that needs to be given in addition to the dose, the patient
would recieve without beeing on continuous hemofiltration. The
relative contribution of extracorporal drug clearance to
overall drug elimination can be demonstrated by mathematical
means.

$$Cl(B) = \frac{A(0)}{AUC} \qquad and \qquad Cl(CAVH) = \frac{A(CAVH)}{AUC}$$

rearranged:

$$AUC = \frac{A(0)}{Cl(B)} \qquad and \qquad AUC = \frac{A(CAVH)}{Cl(CAVH)}$$

both formulas combined and assuming the Cl(CAVH)
beeing equal to the ultrafiltrate flow rate (UF)
the equation transforms to:

$$A(CAVH) = A(0) \times \frac{UF}{Cl(B)}$$

if we divide that formula by A(0), we get the
fraction of the dose removed by CAVH
(Fr(CAVH) = A(CAVH)/A(0))

$$Fr(CAVH) = \frac{UF}{Cl(B)} \qquad\qquad (equation\ 1)$$

(Abbreviations: A(0) = amount of a drugs dose systemically
available, A(CAVH) = amount of drug eliminated by CAVH within
an infinite period of time, AUC = the area under the plasma
level - time curve within the same time period, Cl(B) = the
total drug clearance, Cl(CAVH) = the extracorporal clearance
of the drug by CAVH, Fr(CAVH) = fraction of the dose removed
by CAVH for a sieving coefficient of 1, UF = Ultrafiltrate
flow rate)

Varying standard pharmacokinetic formulas (see above) it
can be shown, that the fraction of the dose of a drug removed
by hemofiltration is related to the drug's clearance by CAVH.
It is however inversely correlated to total body clearance,
which is in anuric patients the nonrenal clearance plus the

drug clearance by hemofiltration (equation 1). As a consequence, the higher the body clearance of a drug in relation to the extracorporal drug clearance, the lower will be the amount of drug and thus the fraction of the dose removed by hemofiltration. If a drug`s total clearance reaches 40 ml/min, thus six times the usual CAVH clearance, the fraction of the dose removed by CAVH is less than 20% and can be regarded as clinically insignificant.

To further illustrate this aspect, the total clearance of the carbapenem antibiotic Imipenem, the extracorporal clearance and the fraction of the Imipenem dose eliminated by arterivenous hemofiltration in two selected patients is depicted in table 1.

Table 1. Impact of CAVH on overall Imipenem elimination in two selected patient with different degrees of renal function. (Cl(B) = total Clearance, Cl(CAVH) = extracorporal clearance by CAVH, Fr(CAVH) = Fraction of the dose eliminated by CAVH)

patient	Cl(B) (ml/min)	Cl(CAVH) (ml/min)	Fr(CAVH)
normal renal function	283	7.1	0.016
acute renal failure	73	4.7	0.062

In the patient with normal renal function, the high total clearance of 283 ml/min results in an insignificant fraction of Imipenem eliminated by CAVH (1.6 %). In the patient with acute renal failure the total clearance is markedly reduced to 73 ml/min; it is however still much higher than the Imipenem clearance via CAVH, leading to a loss of Imipenem by this route of only 6.2 % of the dose.

In patients with normal renal function almost identical pharmacokinetic properties of Imipenem and Cilastatin have been reported (Norrby et al. 1984, Drusano and Standiford 1985). As shown in fig. 2, in critically ill patients with acute renal failure the mean plasma level-time profile of Cilastatin, which is exclusively eliminated by renal routes, is different from that of Imipenem. The elimination half life of Cilastatin is more prolonged than that of Imipenem, since the latter drug is also eliminated via metabolism in the plasma. This difference in kinetic properties of Cilastatin in relation to Imipenem in acute renal failure leads to a relatively and absolutely higher elimination of Cilastatin by hemofiltration.

Table 2. Impact of CAVH on overall Cilastatin elimination in two selected patients with different degrees of renal impairment. For abbreviations see table 1

patient	Cl(B) (ml/min)	Cl(CAVH) (ml/min)	Fr(CAVH)
normal renal function	205	5.1	0.025
acute renal failure	11	6.5	0.59

As shown in table 2 the loss of Cilastatin in a patient with normal renal function is negligible accounting for only 2.5 % of the dose. With renal failure Cilastatin becomes a low clearance drug, the total clearance, beeing only 11 ml/min in that patient. Consequently, the fraction of the dose removed by continuous hemofiltration is as high as 60%.

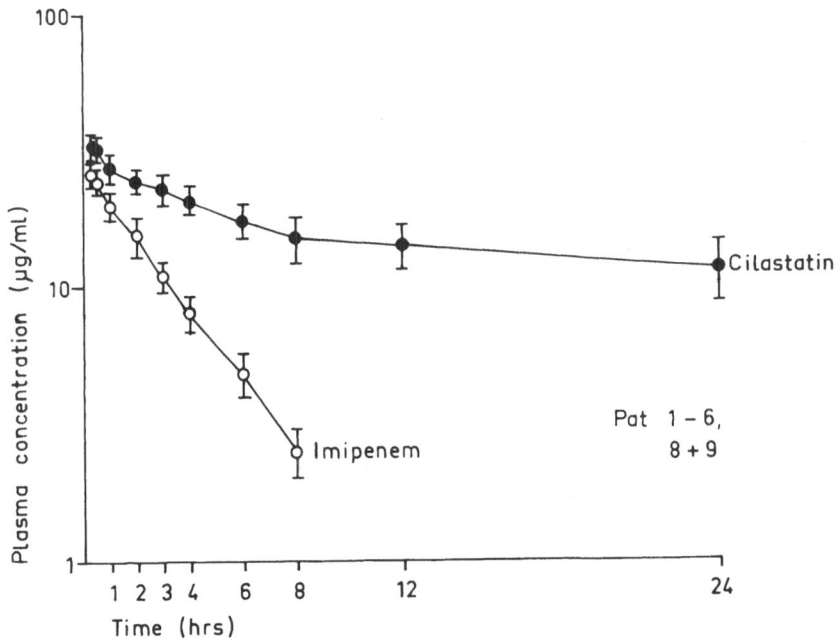

Figure 2. Plasma level-time profile of Imipenem and Cilastatin (500/500 mg i.v.) in 8 critically ill patients with acute renal failure during CAVH (Keller et al. 1989).

Sieving and Drug Protein Binding

The assumptions made here (equation 1), however, are not
sufficient for they do not take into account the protein
binding and drug membrane interactions, which may further
reduce drug movement across the filter membrane. The molecular
cut off of the most frequently used polysulfon membranes of 10
thousand Dalton guarentees the free movement of drug molecules, because virtually all drugs in clinical use have a
molecular weight below this value. The fraction of the drug,
however, bound to macromolecules like albumin will not
traverse the membrane. Thus the plasma protein binding, which
may account for up to 99% of a drug may further limit the
eliminative capacity of hemofiltration. The retention of drugs
by the filter membrane can be expressed as the sieving
coefficient, which relates the drug concentration in the
ultrafiltrate to that in the arterial line (Golper et al.
1986). Thus the lower the drug concentration in the ultrafiltrate in comparison to that in the arterial line, the lower
the sieving coefficient will be. As could be shown by Golper
et al. sieving depends mainly on drug protein binding and not
on drug-protein-membrane interactions.

For example, with a protein binding of less than 20%
(Reeves et al. 1983, Drusano et al. 1985), ultrafiltrate and
plasma levels of Imipenem were identical leading to a sieving
coefficient of approximately 1 in our study (fig.3a). The
plasma protein binding of Cilastatin, however, is reported to
approximate 40 % (Gibson et al. 1985), which may explain the
ultrafiltrate levels beeing significantly lower than the
plasma levels of the drug. The mean sieving value measured
0.77 in our patients (fig.3b).

If an assay to measure drug concentrations in blood and
ultrafiltrate is not available one might consider the plasma
protein binding of a drug in uremic patients (Bennett et al
1983, Vanholder et al. 1988) as the major restriction for drug
movement across the filter membrane; the sieving coefficient
in equation 2 can be sustituted for the free fraction of the
drug (Fr(free)) in plasma. To get an estimate of the amount of
drug actually eliminated by continuous hemofiltration we can
multiply the already calculated values (by equation 1) with
the sieving coefficient or, if not available, with the free
fraction of the drug in uremic plasma (see equation 2).

$$Fr(CAVH) = \frac{UF}{Cl(B)} \times S \text{ (or } Fr(free)) \qquad \text{(equation 2)}$$

(Fr(CAVH) = fraction of the drug dose removed by CAVH, UF =
ultrafiltrate flow rate, Cl(B) = total drug clearance, S =
sieving coefficient, Fr(free) = fraction of the drug not bound
to serum proteins)

In table 3, the total drug clearance (column 2) in renal
failure (review Bennett et al. 1983) plus the estimated
maximal CAVH clearance (= usual ultrafiltration rate) and that
ultrafiltration rate are set into relation for some important
drugs frequently used in intensive care patients. The theoretically estimated maximal amount of drug removed by hemo-

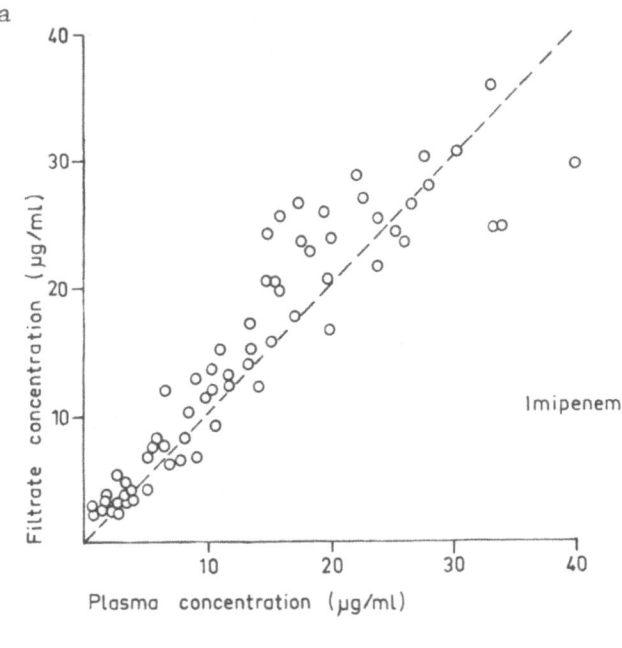

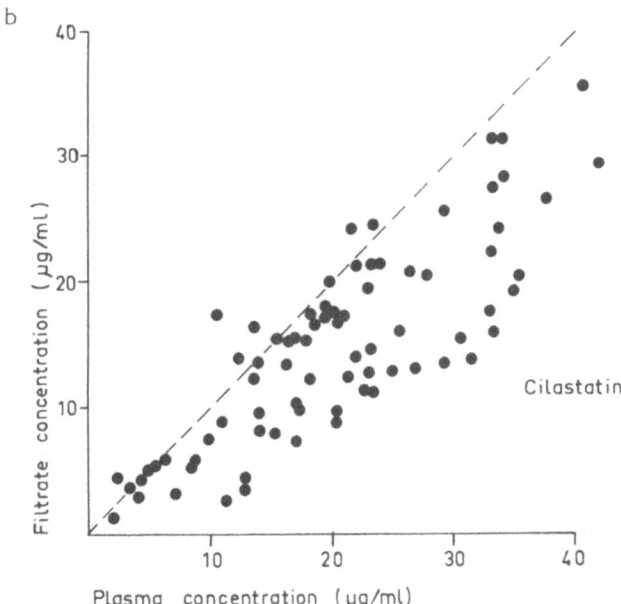

Figure 3 a,b. Relation between Imipenem(3a)/Cilastatin(3b)
concentrations in the arterial line of the extracorporal
system and the drug concentrations found in the ultrafiltrate.

Table 3. Basic pharmacokinetic parameters of some drugs, frequently used in the critically ill. Estimation of the fraction of the dose eliminated by CAVH. Cl(B) = total clearance, Cl(CAVH) = extracorporal clearance by CAVH, Fr(free) = fraction of the drug not bound to macromolecules, Fr(CAVH) = fraction of the dose eliminated by CAVH, corrected for the protein binding and sieving of the drug, eq. = equation

DRUG	Cl(B) in renal failure -(ml/min)-	Cl(CAVH)	Result from eq.1 UF/Cl(B)	Fr(free)	Fr(CAVH)
DOBUTAMIN	4000	6	0.0015	1	0.0015
PHENYTOIN	130	6	0.05	0.25	0.01
THEOPHYLLIN	60	6	0.1	0.6	0.06
DIGOXIN	21	6	0.29	0.7	0.20
DIGITOXIN	9	6	0.66	0.05	0.03
TOBRAMYCIN	12	6	0.5	1	0.50
VANCOMYCIN	8	6	0.75	1	0.75

filtration (Cl(CAVH)/Cl(B), see equation 1) is negligible for Dobutamin beeing far below 1%, because of its extraordinarily high total clearance of approximately 4000 ml/min (Kates and Leier 1978). In the case of Digoxin, Tobramycin, Digitoxin and Vancomycin, however, supplementing the dose for the loss by continuous hemofiltration might be nessesary.

Applying equation 2 the finally estimated fraction of the dose removed by CAVH (table 3) will be further decreased for phenytoin, theophyllin, digoxin and particularly for the highly protein bound digitoxin. Tobramycin and Vancomycin, however, exhibit still significant elimination by CAVH with the need for a change in dosing schedules. For aminoglykosides and Vancomycin these estimations were confirmed by Zarowitz et al. (1986) and Lau et al. (1987), who found significant elimination of these substances in critically ill patients on CAVH.

The Volume of Distribution

For the estimation of the apparent volume of distribution it is assumed that the body is a homogenous reservoir
of water and that the drug distributes freely. The distribution volume of a drug is usually considered a major
determinant of its ease to be eliminated by extracorporal
measures. Drugs with low tissue binding, i.e. low volume of
distribution, will lead to a significant portion of the drug
remaining in the central compartment. There the drug is easily
accessible in the bloodstream for elimination by extracorporal
routes but also by physiological pathways. Drugs with
significant tissue binding, i.e. a large distribution volume,
however, are accessible in the circulation for extracorporal
elimination only to a very limited extent. The assumption,
however, that a drug needs to be in the circulation to be
eliminated, holds true for nearly all cases for the physiological pathways of drug elimination as well. Thus, not the
drugs volume of distribution but the competition between the
extracorporal and the physiological elimination route (as
shown in equation 2) determines the impact of hemofiltration
for overall drug elimination. In case of a low clearance by
physiological routes, a large volume of distribution does not
lead automatically to insignificant extracorporal elimination.
When elimination by extracorporal measures, however, super-
venes physiological elimination of a drug with high volume of
distribution, the elimination by the low ultrafiltration rate
will take a long time. That makes CAVH unsuitable for the
treatment of drug intoxications. It does however not exclude
the necessity of adjusting the dose for CAVH for drugs with
high volume of distribution.

CONCLUSIONS

To estimate the fraction of the dose of a particular drug
removed by CAVH one should divide the mean ultrafiltration
rate by the total clearance, consisting of the residual body
clearance (taken from the literature, reviewed by Bennett et
al. 1983) and the ultrafiltration rate. The derived value
should be multiplied with the sieving coefficient (which can
be calculated from measured drug levels in plasma and ultrafiltrate) or, if not available, should be multiplied with the
unbound fraction of the drug (taken from the literature, for
example Vanholder et al. 1988). The result is the fraction of
the dose lost by continuous hemofiltration (eq. 2). If this is
below 20%, dosage adjustment may not be needed; if it is
above that value additional dosing should be considered, and
blood level monitoring of the drug is recommended.

These pharmacokinetic considerations do not supplement
sophisticated pharmacokinetic studies in patients on CAVH;
they give, however, some guidelines for the drug therapy as
long as such studies are not available. Drugs which are
calculated to be eliminated to a very limited extend (for
example below 10 % of the dose) may not need to be investigated by expensive pharmacokinetic studies. For estimating the
impact of CAVH on drug elimination only few clinical and
pharmacokinetic information like renal function, ultrafiltration rate, total drug clearance and sieving coefficient (or
the protein binding of the drug) are needed.

In many cases estimations by equation 2 will be particularly valuable to realize insignificant drug elimination by CAVH. If a drug elimination higher than 20% of the dose is calculated, however, drug therapy should be monitored by measurement of drug levels in blood or plasma. Considering this limitation, the principles discussed may be transferred as well to CAVH related treatment modalities like venovenous hemofiltration or continuous arteriovenous hemodialysis.

REFERENCES

Bennett W.M., Aronoff G.R., Morrison G., Golper T.A., Pulliam J., Wolfson M., Singer I., 1983, Drug prescribing in renal failure: Dosing guidelines for adults, Am. J. Kidney. Dis., 3: 155.

Bodenham A., Shelly M.P., Park G.R., 1988, The altered pharmacokinetics and pharmacodynamics of drugs commonly used in critically ill patients, Clin. Pharmacokin., 14: 347.

Bozkurt F., Hörl W.H., 1987, Bedeutung der kontinuierlichen arteriovenösen Hämofiltration (CAVH) und arteriovenösen Hämodiafiltration (AV-HDF) in der Intensivtherapie, Intensivmed., 24: 248.

Drusano G.L., Standiford H.C., 1985, Pharmacokinetic profile of Imipenem/Cilastatin in normal volunteers, Am. J. Med., 78: 47.

Gibson T.P., Demetriades J.L., Bland J.A., 1985, Imipenem/Cilastatin: Pharmacokinetic profile in renal insufficiency, Am. J. Med., 78 (suppl. 6 a): 54.

Golper T.A., Pulliam J., Bennett W.M., 1985, Removal of therapeutic drugs by continuous arteriovenous hemofiltration, Arch. Int. Med., 145: 1651.

Golper T.A., Saad A.M.A., Morris C.D., 1986, Gentamycin and Phenytoin sieving through hollow fiber polysulfone hemofilters, Kidney Int., 30: 937.

Hilt H., Keller F., 1987, Elimination von Pharmaka durch Hämofiltration, Anästh. Intensivther. Notfallmed., 22: 278.

Kates R.E., Leier C.V., 1987, Dobutamine pharmacokinetics in severe heart failure, Clin. Pharmacol. Ther., 24: 537.

Keller E., Fecht H., Böhler J., Schollmeyer P., 1989, Single dose kinetics of Imipenem Cilastatin during continuous arteriovenous hemofiltration in intensive care patients, Nephr. Dial. and Transplant., (submitted).

Kramer P., Wigger W., Rieger J., Mattheai D., Scheler F., 1977, Arteriovenous hemofiltration : a new and simple method for treatment of overhydrated patients resistant to diuretics, Klin. Wochenschr., 55: 1121.

Lau A.H., Kronfol N.O., John E., 1987, Increased vancomycin elimination with continuous hemofiltration, Trans. Am. Soc. Artif. Intern. Organs., 33: 772.

Norrby S.R., Rogers J.D., Ferber F., Jones K.H., Zachei A.G., Weidner L.L., Demetriades J.L., Gravellese D.A., Hsieh Y.K., 1984, Disposition of radiolabeled Imipenem and Cilastatin in normal human volunteers, Antimicrob. Agents. Chemother., 26: 707.

Reeves D.S., Chapman S.T., Davies A.J., Ferber V.F., Rogers J.D., 1983, Human pharmacokinetics of N-Formimidoyl thienamycin alone and in combination with a dehydropeptidase inhibitor (MK 791) and probenecid. In: Spitzy KH, Karrer K eds., Proceedings of the thirteens International congress of Chemotherapy. Vienna, Austria, Vol 3, part 95: 30.

Stevens P.E., Riley B., Davies S.P., Gower P.E., Brown E.A., Kox W., 1988, Continuous arteriovenous hemodialysis in critically ill patients, Lancet 2: 150.

Vanholder R., Landschoot N.V., De Smed R., Schoots A., Ringoir S., 1988, Drug protein binding in chronic renal failure: Evaluation of nine drugs, Kidney Int., 33: 996.

Zarowitz B.J., Anandan J.V., Dumler F., Jayashankar J., Levin N., 1986, Continuous arteriovenous hemofiltration of aminoglykoside antibiotics in critically ill patients. J. Clin. Pharmacol., 26: 686.

THE BIOLOGY OF THE PERITONEAL MEMBRANE

DURING CHRONIC PERITONEAL DIALYSIS

Henri A. Verbrugh, M.D., PhD.

Laboratory for Microbiology, University of Utrecht Medical
School, 59 Catharijnesingel, 3511 GG, Utrecht
The Netherlands

INTRODUCTION

The peritoneal cavity is lined by a membrane consisting of a single
layer of mesothelial cells resting on a thin basement membrane; underneath
the mesothelial cell layer loose connective tissues contain the capillaries
that are essential for dialysis. The mesothelial cell layer is rather unique,
it is of mesodermal origin and covers the large body cavities. Morphologic
studies have shown that mesothelial cells have microvilli on their apical
surface and that their surfaces are covered with slippery glycocalix[1,2].

The mesothelium is thought to perform crucial functions in the transport of water and solutes across the peritoneal membrane as well as providing a slippery, non-adhesive and non-thrombogenic, surface that allows for
smooth motility of internal organs[3,4]. Chronic peritoneal dialysis (CPD) has
been associated with alternations in the peritoneal membrane. Mesothelial
cells tend to lose their surface microvilli and show a widening of intercellular spaces or become completely detached from the basement membrane at
several sites; in addition, there is fibrosis underneath the mesothelium[5,6].
Bacterial peritonitis seems to augment and accelerate such changes, which
may be correlated with altered rates of water and solute transport during
CPD[6,7]. However, little is known about the underlying mechanisms that lead
to membrane pathology. We studied the effects of CPD fluids and of bacterial
products on the morphology and viability of human mesothelial cells in vitro.
The results show that mesothelial cells are lysed upon prolonged contact with
CPD fluids. Likewise, staphylococcal species may release exoproducts that
directly kill human mesothelial cells.

MATERIAL AND METHODS

Mesothelial cells

Human mesothelial cells were isolated from pieces of omentum wasted
during abdominal surgery according to techniques modified from Nicholson et
al.[4] and Wu et al.[8] . The cells were cultured in fibronectin-coated polysty-
rene flasks using medium M199 (Gibco Europe, Breda, Holland) with added hydro-
cortisone sodium succinate (1 μg/ml), fetal calf serum (10%) and antibiotics
(gentamicin + vancomycin); the cells were grown as monolayers in a 37°C,
fully humidified, 5% CO_2 cabinet. In some experiments mesothelial cells were
grown in tissue culture chamber-slides (Lab-Tek, Miles Sci., Naperville, ILL,
U.S.A.).

Light microscopy

The morphology of the mesothelial cell monolayers was studied using Giemsa-stained preparations of control- and treated cells in the chamber-slides. The identity of the mesothelial cells was regularly checked by immunofluorescent staining techniques for cytokeratins and for factor VIII related surface antigen using monoclonal antibodies (Dakopatts, Denmark).

Challenge fluids

Fresh CPD fluids were obtained at all available glucose concentrations from B. Braun Melsungen AG (Melsungen, FRG), Fresenius AG (Bad Homburg, FRG) and Travenol GMBH (München, FRG). Effluent fluids were obtained from non-infected patients undergoing CAPD after various dwell times. Supernates from overnight cultures of seven strains of Staphylococcus aureus and of 29 strains of S. epidermidis were obtained by centrifugation (1600g for 15 minutes) and filter-sterilization; mesothelial cell culture medium without antibiotics was used for bacterial growth.

Cytotoxicity Assay

Mesothelial cell damage was assayed by a ^{51}Cr-release assay[9]. Mesothelial cells were radiolabelled with ^{51}Chromium as sodium chromate (Amersham, UK) and seeded into 96 well flatbottom microtiter trays (Nunclon, Gibco Europe) and incubated overnight. Washed, radiolabelled cell monolayers were exposed to challenge fluids for indicated time periods and, subsequently, sampled for the amount of radiolabel released into the supernatant fluid by gamma-counting. The extent of mesothelial cell lysis is given as a percent ^{51}Cr-release after correction for spontaneous release of the ^{51}Cr from control wells incubated with fresh growth medium. Maximum ^{51}Cr-release was determined in wells treated with 1% Triton X-100[9].

RESULTS

Mesothelial cells formed confluent monolayers with typical "cobblestone" appearance; individual cells had large nuclei and one or more nucleoli (not shown). The identity of mesothelial cells was confirmed by the presence of intracellular cytoskeleton that stained with antibody against human cytokeratin[8]. The cells did not carry the factor VIII related surface antigen. Incubation of mesothelial cell monolayers with fresh CPD fluids resulted in profound morphologic changes: cells were found to retract and shrink, showed signs of vacuolization of the cytoplasm and pyknosis of their nuclei, and upon prolonged incubation dissapeared from the monolayer.

Table 1. Lysis of Cultured Human Mesothelial Cells by Peritoneal Dialysis Fluids

Peritoneal Dialysis Fluids[b] from	% ^{51}Cr-release from mesothelial cells after	
	4 hours	18 hours
B. Braun	5(0-16)[a]	61(40-93)
Fresenius	7(3-10)	54(42-66)
Travenol	59(52-69)[c]	60(50-83)

[a] mean (range) based on at least five separate experiments.
[b] 1.5% glucose (Braun & Fresenius), 1.36% glucose (Travenol).
[c] p<0.001 compared to Braun or Fresenius.

Cell damage could accurately and reproducibly be quantitated by the release of ^{51}Cr from radiolabelled monolayers. All CPD fluids induced a >50% release of ^{51}Cr after 18h incubation indicating extensive structural damage to the cells; CPD fluids from Travenol but not from Braun or Fresenius induced >50% cytotoxicity within 4h incubation (Table 1). CPD fluids were cytotoxic regardless of their glucose content (data not shown). Similarly, neutralisation of CPD fluid pH to 7.3 did reduce but not abolish their cyto-toxicity for mesothelial cells. Taken together these results would indicate that hypertonicity alone or low pH alone may not be responsible for the observed toxicity of CPD fluids. To further study the osmotic- and acid to-lerance of mesothelial cells increasing concentrations (up to 10%) of glucose were added to culture medium and to the same medium acidified to pH 5.5. At pH 7.3 mesothelial cells tolerated 18 h incubation in medium containing up to 2% glucose; higher levels of glucose induced ^{51}Cr-release. At pH 5.5 glucose tolerance was reduced to a 1% maximum (data not shown). Acid medium without added glucose did not induce ^{51}Cr-release. Effluent fluids collected from non-infected patients after 4-6h dwell time did not induce ^{51}Cr-release from mesothelial cell monolayers. In four patients effluent samples were drawn earlier which revealed complete neutralisation of CPD fluid cytotoxi-city after 15 to 120 minutes of dwell in the peritoneal cavity (data not shown).

Supernates from 4/7 (58%) S. aureus cultures were highly toxic for mesothelial cells. Likewise, addition of viable, but not of heatkilled, cells of a cytotoxin-producing strain induced >80% ^{51}Cr-release after 18h (Figure 1). In contrast, only 4/29 (14%) S. epidermidis culture supernates induced cytotoxicity (p<0.01).

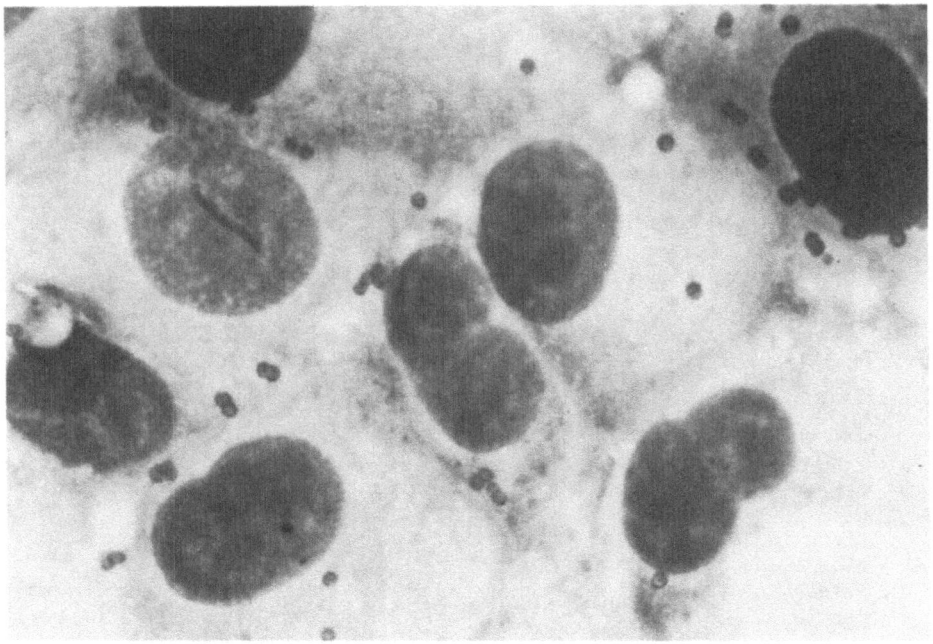

Fig. 1 Giemsa-stained monolayer of human mesothelial cells after 18 h incu-bation with heat-killed S. aureus. Note intact cobblestone morphology of the monolayer with adherent cocci. (magnification, x 1,000).

DISCUSSION

The results of this study show that the currently available CPD fluids are cytotoxic for human mesothelial cells in vitro. In addition, exoproducts from staphylococci, especially S. aureus, may contain cytotoxins that irreversibly damage mesothelial cells. Previous studies by our group[10] and other investigators[11] have indicated that CPD fluids block the activition of the human complement system and decrease the bactericidal activity fo human phagocytes. During the dwell time the cytotoxic potential of CPD fluids is lost within two hours. However, it is reasonable to suggest that repeated exposures to toxic CPD fluids may, in time, lead to permanent changes in the morphology and biology of mesothelial cells. High concentrations of glucose have been shown to induce DNA damage in human endothelial cells[12] . In addition, mesothelial cells can be stimulated to produce various mediators of inflammation and produce collagen and other protein used in the structuring of the submesothelial layers[13,14,15]. Repeated exposure to toxic stimuli either from CPD fluids or from bacteria during episodes of peritonitis may, therefore, indirectly alter the submesothelial tissues as well as the mesothelial cells themselves. Taken together these data further stress the need to develop new recipes for CPD fluids that take into account their compatibility with host tissues. The ability of staphylococci to produce cytotoxins for human mesothelial cells is not surprising. Staphylococci, especially S. aureus, produce a wide variety of potentially toxic proteins that may interfere with cell function or viability[16]. The membrane-damaging toxins such as α-toxin and δ-toxin would be prime candidates to exert toxic effects upon mesothelial cells; preliminary results indicate that α-toxin in the supernates of the S. aureus cultures is indeed partly responsible. S. epidermidis supernates were less likely to contain cytotoxins for mesothelial cells which correlates with their known reduced, but not absent, capacity to produce exotoxins when compared to S. aureus[17] . Our observation that adherence of inactivated staphylococci to mesothelial cells is relatively innocuous indicates that staphylococcal species induce mesothelial damage primarly by secreting exo-toxins.

REFERENCES

1. R. S. Cunningham, The physiology of the serous membrane, Physiol. Rev. 6:242-277 (1926).
2. P. M. Andrews and K. R. Porter, The ultrastructural morphology and possible functional significance of mesothelial microvilli, Anat. rec. 177:409-426 (1974).
3. G. E. Digenis, S. Rabinovich, A. Medline, H. Rodella, G. Wu, and D. G. Oreopoulos, Electron microscopic study of the peritoneal kinetics of iron dextran during peritoneal dialysis in the rabbit, Nephron. 37:108-112 (1984).
4. L. J. Nicholson, J. M. F. Clarke, R. M. Pittilo, S. J. Machin, and N. Woolf, The mesothelial cell as a non-thrombogenic surface, Thromb. Haemostas. 37:108-112 (1984).
5. N. Di Paolo, G. Sacchi, M. De Mia, et al., Morphology of the peritoneal membrane during continuous ambulatory peritoneal dialysis, Nephron. 44:204-211 (1986).
6. J. W. Dobbie and M. A. Zaki, The ultrastructure of the parietal peritoneum in normal and uraemic man and in patients on CAPD. In: "Frontiers in peritoneal dialysis"J. F. Maher and J. F. Winchester, ed., Rich & Assoc., New York (1986).
7. C. Verger, A. Luger, H. L. Moore, and K. D. Nolph, Acute changes in peritoneal morphology and transport properties with infectious peritonitis and mechanical injury, Kidney Int. 23:823-831 (1983).
8. Y. J. Wu, L. M. Parker, N. E. Binder, et al, The mesothelial keratins: a new family of cytoskeletal proteins identified in cultured mesothelial cells and nonkeratinizing epithelia. Cell. 31:693-703 (1982).

9. P. J. Romano, Cytolytic assays for soluble antigens, in: "Manual of clinical laboratory immunology", N. R. Rose, H. Friedman, J. L. Fahey, ed., ASM, Washington DC (1986).

10. H. A. Verbrugh, R. P. Verkooijen, J. Verhoef, P. L. Oe, J. van der Meulen, Defective complement-mediated opsonization and lysis of bacteria in commercial peritoneal dialysis solutions, in: "Frontiers in peritoneal dialysis", J. F. Maher, J. F. Winchester, ed., Rich & Assoc., New York (1986).

11. A. K. Duwe, S. I. Vas, and J. W. Weatherheard, Effects of composition of peritoneal dialyis fluid on chemiluminescence, phagocytosis, and bactericidal activity in vitro, Infect. Immun.33:130-135 (1981).

12. M. Lorenzi, D. F. Montisano, and S. Toledo, High glucose induces DNA damage in cultured human endothelial cells, Barrieux. J. Clin. Invest. 77:322-325 (1986).

13. M. C. Coene, C. Solheid, M. Claeys, and A. G. Herman, Prostaglandin procuction by cultured mesothelial cells, Arch. Int. Pharmacodyn. 249:316-318 (1981).

14. J. O. Cantor, M. Willhite, B. A. Bray, S. Keller, I. Mandl, and G. M. Turino, Synthesis of crosslinked elastin by a mesothelial cell culture (42269), Proc. Soc. Exp. Biol. Med. 181:387-391 (1986).

15. W. Harvey and P. L. Amlot, Collagen production by human mesothelial cells in vitro, J. Pathol. 139:337-347 (1983).

16. M. Rogolsky, Nonenteric toxins of Staphylococcus aureus, Microbiol. Rev. 43:320-360 (1979).

17. C. G. Gemmell, Virulence characteristics of Staphylococcus epidermidis, J. Med. Microbiol. 22:289-291 (1986).

LYMPHATIC ABSORPTION DURING PERITONEAL DIALYSIS

Karl D. Nolph, M.D.

University of Missouri Health Sciences Center
Dalton Research Center, and VA Hospital
Columbia, MO

INTRODUCTION

In recent years, our group has published several reviews of the literature on peritoneal lymphatics[1-2] and studies of peritoneal lymphatics during peritoneal dialysis in rats[3-5] and in humans.[6-7] Herein I will summarize some of the major points in those publications.

GENERAL CONCEPTS

On the undersurface of the diaphragm there are large intercellular gaps between adjacent mesothelial cells. These stoma are open during diaphragmatic relaxation and close during diaphragmatic contraction. Beneath these stoma balloon like endings (lacunae) of diaphragmatic lymphatics are found. Flap like extensions of lymphatic endothelial cells form valve like openings into the lacunae beneath the stoma.

Although hypotonic fluids may be absorbed into peritoneal capillary venules, it is likely that high intraperitoneal isoosmotic solutions are absorbed mainly by the subdiaphragmatic system. Because of the large mean pore diameters of this system, dissolved solutes of even high molecular weight are swept along with this absorption by convection. Absorption of molecules above 20,000 daltons in molecular weight may be exclusively by this system without molecular size discrimination. Numerous studies now suggest that molecules above 20,000 daltons in molecular weight have similar fractional absorptions from intraperitoneal solutions. Such absorption usually take place with little or no change in the concentration of the larger molecular weight substance in the solution again compatible with convective mechanisms for absorption.

There is some question as to whether fluids and high molecular weight substances can move directly into the peritoneal tissues at other sites with eventual movement into venules or lymphatics. Further work is needed to prove whether the pathway for the absorption of isoosmotic fluids and high molecular weight substances from the peritoneal cavity is entirely by the subdiaphragmatic system.

RAT STUDIES

Techniques have been developed to measure lymphatic outflow from the peritoneal cavity. These are based on the assumption that the absorption of a high molecular weight marker would be entirely by convective mechanisms through the subdiaphragmatic lymphatics or other convective pathways into lymphatics. Solutions are instilled into the peritoneal cavity containing a large molecular weight marker such as albumin. The clearance of the marker from the peritoneal cavity is assumed to represent a close estimate of lymphatic flow. In our rat model, we have demonstrated lymphatic flow rates averaging 4.7 ml per hour during peritoneal dialysis using very hypertonic exchanges (15% dextrose). Fifty four percent of the actual transcapillary ultrafiltration generated can be absorbed by the peritoneal lymphatics over a six hour exchange.

Documentation of the importance of lymphatic absorption also alters our understanding of the kinetics of ultrafiltration. For example, the peak of intraperitoneal volume during a hypertonic exchange is not at osmotic equilibrium but at the point where transcapillary ultrafiltration equals lymphatic reabsorption. Because the ultrafiltrate is low in electrolytes, osmotic equilibrium and even a hypoosmolar phase of dialysate is produced before glucose equilibrium. Because of the relative importance of the glucose sieving coefficient in determining transmembrane osmotic pressure, some transcapillary ultrafiltration continues even during the hypoosmolar phase. At eventual glucose equilibrium and osmotic equilibrium, the absorption rate becomes equal to that of lymphatic absorption and similar to the absorption rate seen with isoosmotic solutions such as Lactated Ringers.

HUMAN STUDIES

Using albumin as a marker, lymphatic absorption rates have been estimated in clinical studies. Ultrafiltration kinetics similar to those seen in a rat model have been demonstrated. The studies suggest that in patients using four 2.5% 2 liter six hour exchanges per day the lymphatic absorption would amount to 82% of the actual daily transcapillary ultrafiltration generated. Drain volumes, urea clearances, and creatinine clearances, would be reduced by 18, 14, and 13% from what they would be without lymphatic absorption.

Studies in children have shown lymphatic absorption rates representing an even higher proportion of transcapillary ultrafiltration. For example, a child demonstrates absorption rates of 10.3 ml/kg body weight compared to 4.4 in adults with four hour 2.5% dextrose exchanges.

MANIPULATIONS OF LYMPHATIC ABSORPTION IN THE RAT

Topical application of cholinergic drugs to the subdiaphragmatic surface is known to narrow or close the subdiaphragmatic stoma during diaphragmatic relaxation. Whether the drug maintains surrounding muscle tone or effects microfilamentary structures in the cells and adjacent tissues is not clear. Studies were carried out in rats with and without neostigmine added to the peritoneal dialysis solutions. With neostigmine, net ultrafiltration was significantly increased using 2.5% dextrose exchanges and two hour cycles. This increase in net ultrafiltration was accounted for by comparable decreases in lymphatic absorption rates as estimated by the absorption of albumin from the peritoneal cavity. Increases in clearances could be accounted for entirely by increases in drain volume. There were no changes in dialysate/plasma concentration ratios of urea creatinine or phosphate.

Phosphatidylcholine is a substrate for the formation of acetylcholine and therefore may have cholinergic effects. Also, it is cationic and may neutralize dense clusters of anionic charges in the stoma area. These anionic charges may repel one another and help keep stoma open. In the rat model, peritoneal dialysis solutions containing phosphatidylcholine were associated with similar decreases in lymphatic absorption and increases in net ultrafiltration as seen with neostigmine.

In additional rat studies, India ink was added to peritoneal dialysis solution with or without phosphatidylcholine. In the absence of phosphatidylcholine, India ink could be seen filling the diaphragmatic lymphatics following sacrifice of the animals post exchange and examination of the diaphragm. On the other hand, with the addition of phosphatidylcholine, the uptake of India ink into the diaphragmatic lymphatics was blocked.

SUMMARY

These studies suggest that lymphatic absorption reduces net ultrafiltration by significant amounts and plays a major role in the overall ultrafiltration kinetics. Intraperitoneal drugs which decrease lymphatic absorption may increase net ultrafiltration, drainage volume, and solute clearances. Decreases in net ultrafiltration with drugs that decrease lymphatic absorption may provide an alternative means to increase net ultrafiltration with less use of hypertonic dextrose exchanges.

REFERENCES

1. R. Khanna, R.A. Mactier, K.D., Nolph, and Z.J. Twardowski, Anatomy of peritoneal cavity lymphatics, Perit Dial Bull 6:113 (1986).

2. R.A. Mactier, R. Khanna, Z.J. Twardowski, and K.D. Nolph, Role of peritoneal cavity lymphatic absorption in peritoneal dialysis, Kidney Int 32:165 (1987).

3. K.D. Nolph, R. Mactier, R. Khanna, Z.J. Twardowski, H. Moore, and T. McGary, The kinetics of ultrafiltration during peritoneal dialysis: The role of lymphatics, Kidney Int 32:219 (1987).

4. R.A. Mactier, R. Khanna, H. Moore, Z.J. Twardowski, and K.D. Nolph, Reduction of lymphatic absorption from the peritoneal cavity with intraperitoneal neostigmine, phosphatidylcholine and other drugs. Peritoneal Dialysis (Proceedings of Third International Course on Peritoneal Dialysis, Vicenza-Italy, 1988) La Greca G., Chiaramonta S., Fabris A., Feriani M., Ronco C., eds. Wichtig Editore, Milano Publishers 41 (1988).

5. R.A. Mactier, R. Khanna, Z.J. Twardowski, H. Moore, and K.D. Nolph, Influence of phosphatidylcholine on lymphatic absorption during peritoneal dialysis in the rat. In press - Perit Dial Internat.

6. R. A. Mactier, R. Khanna, Z.T. Twardowski, H. Moore, and K.D. Nolph, Contribution of lymphatic absorption to loss of ultrafiltration and

solute clearances in continuous ambulatory peritoneal dialysis. J Clin Invest 80:1311 (1987).

7.   R.A. Mactier, R. Khanna, H. Moore, J. Russ, K.D. Nolph, and T. Groshong, Kinetics of peritoneal dialysis in children: Role of lymphatics. Kidney Int 34:82 (1988).

CAPD WITH BICARBONATE SOLUTION

M. Feriani and G. La Greca

Dept. of Nephrology, St. Bortolo Hospital
36100 Vicenza, Italy

One of the major results achieved with CAPD is the good correction of metabolic acidosis and the maintenance of a satisfactory acid-base status. This fact is confirmed by an average plasma bicarbonate concentration in patients on CAPD ranging between 22 and 25 mMol/l. This result appears to be stable over time and acid-base fluctuations, typical of intermittent treatments, are not observed. The steadiness of acid-base status depends on the continuous infusion of buffers in absence of significant losses into dialysate of bicarbonate and permits a good stability of blood gases and ventilation.

Bicarbonate was initially used in 1964 by Boen in peritoneal dialysis fluid (1), but it was soon replaced by lactate, when it was found that calcium carbonate precipitated and the solution became alkaline during autoclaving. In fact, solutions containing bicarbonate, calcium and glucose are difficult to prepare, sterilize and store. So as alkaline agents lactate and subsequently in Europe acetate were introduced.

GENERAL ACID-BASE CONCEPTS IN CAPD

During dialysis, the actual correction of acid-base imbalance depends on several factors (2):
1) the quantity of buffer really gained by the patient;
2) the patient's ability to metabolize the incoming buffer load;
3) the loss of bicarbonate and organic anions into the dialysate.

The influx of buffer and its metabolism must generate enough bicarbonate to replace the bicarbonate and the other alkaline equivalents losses and the buffers utilized to neutralize the "fixed acids" generated by metabolism.

LACTATE AND ACETATE UNPHYSIOLOGY

The buffers currently utilized in CAPD, that is lactate and in a very small percentage of cases acetate, pose metabolic problems, have important side effects and lower the dialysate pH.

Metabolic problems

Lactate and acetate must be fully metabolized to generate bicarbonate. In case of scarce or slowed metabolism (lactic acidosis, diabetes, Addison's disease, alcoholism, overload of buffers and, perhaps, in uremia) the existing acidosis may even worsen.

For example, as suggested by Dixon (3) and by our group (4) lactate infused with dialysis may sometimes be not fully metabolized, possibly causing deterioration of the body buffer pool. However, many problems linked to its metabolism have still to be clarified.

Side effects

Lactate and acetate, which are not inert, present some systemic effects. Both of them are peripheral vasodilators, have effects on myocardial contractility, are directly responsible for a reduction of blood pressure and are belie-ved - mainly acetate - to have a role in dyslipidemia of dialyzed patients.

pH of the solutions

Dialysis solutions containing lactate or acetate have a pH ranging from 5.0 to 6.0 in order to avoid glucose carame-lizing. The low pH of the solutions, the buffer action per se and the hyperosmolality of the solution could be the cause of the initial peritoneal vasodilation. The low pH of the solution, even if rapidly corrected by bicarbonate diffusion from blood into the dialysate, could damage the biological membrane and perhaps trigger an immunological response.

The initial effect of the entry of the buffers into the blood is an acidification, because it changes the rate undissociate/dissociate, increasing the amount of salt, thereby liberating a quantity of free H+. The buffer effect starts when metabolization begins.

For all these reasons bicarbonate should be the preferred buffer; bicarbonate, in fact, does not need any metabolization, renders the pH of dialysate physiological, does not present any known side effect and particularly should not stimulate any immunological response of the biological membrane.

BICARBONATE CHEMICAL BACKGROUND

In hemodialysis, bicarbonate dialysis is routinely done both with a single-pass system which continuously mixes an acid and a basic solution and with a recirculated system in which the mixing has to be done just before use. In peritoneal dialysis, the problem is much more complex, mainly because the solutions are performed, sterilized by autoclave at high temperature and stored for a long period, usually longer than 12 months. During autoclaving, calcium carbonate precipitates:

$$NaHCO_3 + CaCl_2 < ----- > CaCO_3 + NaCl + HCl \qquad (1)$$

For these reasons, up to now, $NaHCO_3$ has been used in PD only as an experimental buffer.

Since early 80's, our group has studied a bicarbonate solution for PD based on chemical laws (5): in fact an high CO_2 content in the solution could guarantee the generation of souble $Ca(HCO_3)_2$, avoiding the precipitation of insoluble $CaCO_3$. In such a case reaction 2 is shifted to the left:

$$Ca(HCO_3)_2 < ----- > CaCO_3 + H_2O + CO_2 \qquad (2)$$

An high adequate CO_2 pressure can be obtained when an acid solution (for example, one containing acetic or lactic acid) reacts with $NaHCO_3$, as shown in reaction 3

$$NaHCO_3 + CH_3COOH < ----- > CH_3COONa + H_2O + CO_2 \qquad (3)$$

So the CO_2 generated shifts reaction 2 to the left and calcium bicarbonate (soluble) is produced while $CaCO_3$ (insoluble) is absent.

Since CO_2 is a gas and therefore volatile, when all the acid (acetic, lactic acid) has been consumed being converted to sodium salt, the fall in the CO_2 content can shift reaction 2 to right and cause precipitation of calcium carbonate. Such a problem can be approached by using two different solutions, one containing bicarbonate, the second calcium plus a small amount of an organic acid, in our experience acetic acid like bicarbonate hemodialysis. These two solutions must be separately prepared, sterilized, stored and must be mixed only few minutes before infusion.

In this system the container must be made of an organic polymer with a low permeability to water vapour and CO_2. Polyethylene and PVC are perferred and are the constituent of the inner foil of commercially available CAPD bags (6).

CLINICAL AND KINETIC STUDIES WITH BICARBONATE CAPD SOLUTIONS

Our experience with bicarbonate PD started in 1984 utilizing an home-made solution prepared in a two-chamber system by pharmacy of our hospital (7). We used this dialysate in 4 patients to clarify the kinetic aspects of the bicarbonate solution and to verify its clinical effectiveness.

Table 1 shows the composition of final dialysate obtained by mixing the acid and the alkaline part. The buffer content of the dialysate was 35 mMoles of bicarbonate plus

5 mMoles of acetate. The final solution was homogenous, stable for more than 24 hours, a period much longer than the utilization time CaCO3 starts precipitating 24 hours after mixing. From a clinical point of view, the solution was well tolerated by the patients; neither abdominal pain nor cloudy effluent occurred.

The patient population and the duration of the trial are depicted in table II.

Table I.   COMPOSITION OF THE PRELIMINARY SOLUTION

Na	=	138 mEq/l	Cl	=	104 mEq/l
K	=	1 mEq/l	HCO3	=	35 mEq/l
Ca	=	4 mEq/l	CH3COO	=	5 mEq/l
Mg	=	1 mEq/l	Glucose	=	16.5 g/l

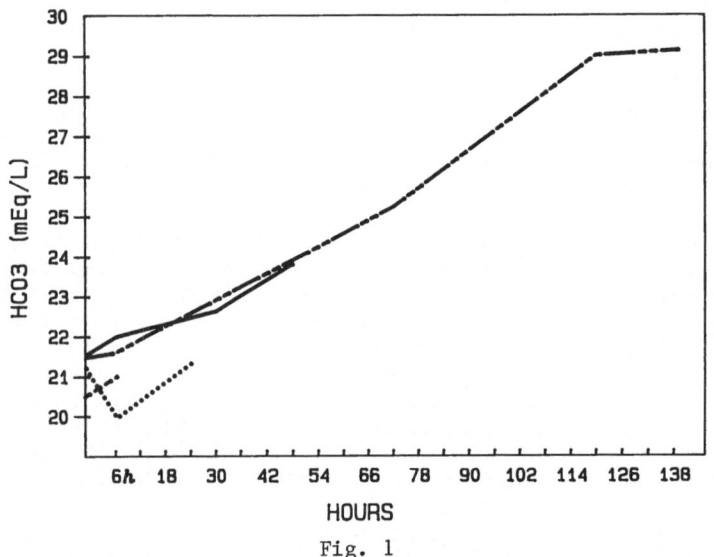

Fig. 1

During the study the bicarbonate blood values increased up to 29 mMol/l in the patient who had the longest treatment, but at this level the slope showed a plateau. This suggested that an equilibrium point does exist indicating that bicarbonate absorption is self limited (figure 1).

Actually the concentration of HCO3 in the dialysate at different dwell time appeared to be linked with the bicarbonate blood levels.
The closest relationship was found after 12 hours dwelltime, when the solution tends to equilibrate with blood (figure 2).

We concluded that bicarbonate CAPD could be performed

through the two chamber bag system and started to look for a factory interested in such an idea.

In April 87 a dialysis solution made by Fresenius became available. The composition of the dialysate was: bicarbonate 27, acetate 3, calcium 1.5, sodium 135 mMol/l.

Table II.   CLINICAL TRIAL

Number of patients	= 4
Dialysis schedules	= 4 x 2 liter-exchanges/day
Duration of the trial	= Patient 1 : 6 hrs (1 exchange)
	Patient 2 : 1 day (4 exchanges)
	Patient 3 : 2 days (8 exchanges)
	Patient 4 : 7 days (28 exchanges)

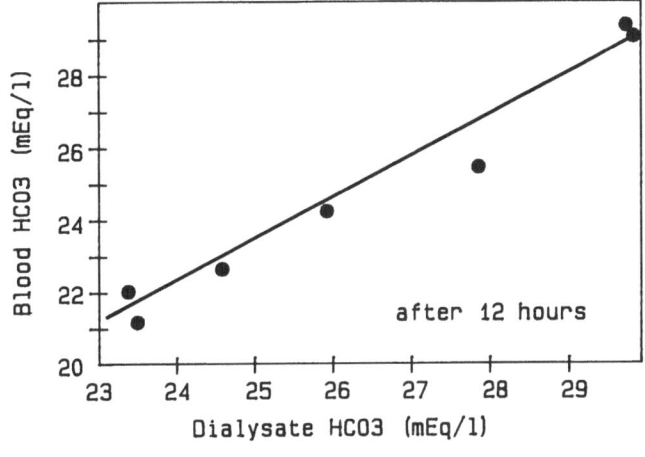

Fig. 2

Table III shows the acid-base status of one patient treated for two months with this new solution.

This patient started with a metabolic acidosis and her pattern didn't change during the treatment. Subsequently a kinetic study was carried out comparing the results obtained with Fresenius bag with those obtained by using our home made solution with 35 mMol/l of bicarbonate.

Figure 3 shows the acid-base kinetic of the Fresenius solution at different dwell-times till 12 hours. Significant changes were seen just after two hours dwell-time: at subsequent observation no further variations were observed. All data are statistically different from basal values but there isn't any difference among different dwell-time. It's very important to point out that during this exchange the mean bicarbonate concentration in arterial blood was 21.4

mMol/l without remarkable deviations from the mean value during all the study. This means that even if the dwell-time is prolonged to 12 hours a gradient of about 5 mMol/l between solution and blood bicarbonate is still maintained.

Table III. LONG TERM STUDY (1 PATIENT 2 MONTHS)
Arterial blood acid-base status

	start	1st month	2nd month
pH	7.33	7.35	7.33
pCO2	37.0	37.7	37.1
HCO3	19.3	20.3	19.0

	pH	pCO2 (mmHg)	HCO3 (mMol/L)	TCO2 (mMol/L)
Basal	7.17 ± 0.04	82.2 ± 7.1	26.9 ± 0.7	29.4 ± 0.8
2h	* 7.32 ± 0.02	* 57.5 ± 1.4	* 25.7 ± 0.4	* 27.4 ± 0.4
4h	* 7.32 ± 0.02	* 56.8 ± 3.5	* 25.6 ± 0.7	* 27.3 ± 0.8
6h	* 7.34 ± 0.03	* 53.3 ± 4.6	* 25.2 ± 0.6	* 26.8 ± 0.7
12h	* 7.33 ± 0.03	* 56.2 ± 2.3	* 26.0 ± 0.9	* 27.7 ± 0.8

* = Students' 't' test significance $p < 0.01$ from basal value

Fig. 3

Figure 4 compares these data with those obtained with the higher bicarbonate concentration at the same HCO3 arterial blood values. Except for the basal values, the points of these slopes do not differ significantly. This means that, after two hour dwell-time, the gradient solution/blood is not dependent on the initial bicarbonate concentration but only on the bicarbonatemia. So being this gradient approximately 5 mMoles in our experiments it seems reasonable to indicate that 30 mMoles of bicarbonate in the dialysate should be enough to reach 25 mMoles of bicarbonate in the arterial blood. Such a high gradient is not quite easily explanable after so long dwell-time. The Donnan's equilibrium could explain only a small quantity of these 5 mMoles.

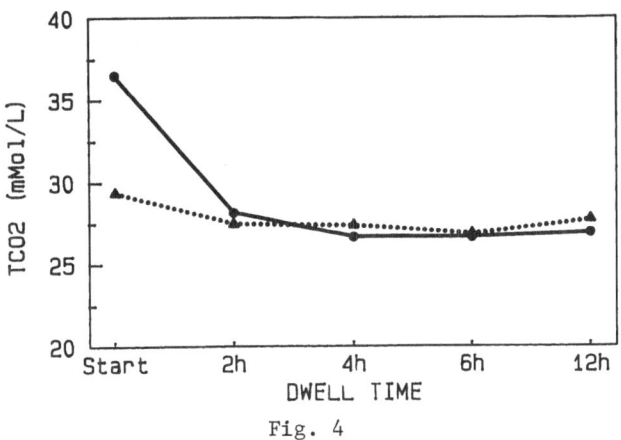

Fig. 4

Furthermore a temptative interpretation could be made by the gradient existing among arterial, peripheral venous and splancnic venous blood (figure 5). The pCO2 levels in the dialysate after 6 hours of dwell-time are always much higher than the arterial blood ones. CO2 in fact is very diffusible and peritoneal membrane does not represent an obstacle to its diffusion. However the dialysate pCO2 is better equilibrated with venous than arterial blood. The blood leaving the mesothelium is supposed to be quite different from the blood leaving, for example, the arm. Actually the slower flux of enteric circulation should make its venous blood more charged of CO2 and consequently with higher levels of HCO3 and a lower pH. The dialysate could equilibrate with this blood.

Figure 6 shows the kinetic of the small quantity of acetate present in the solution. The buffer disappearance is

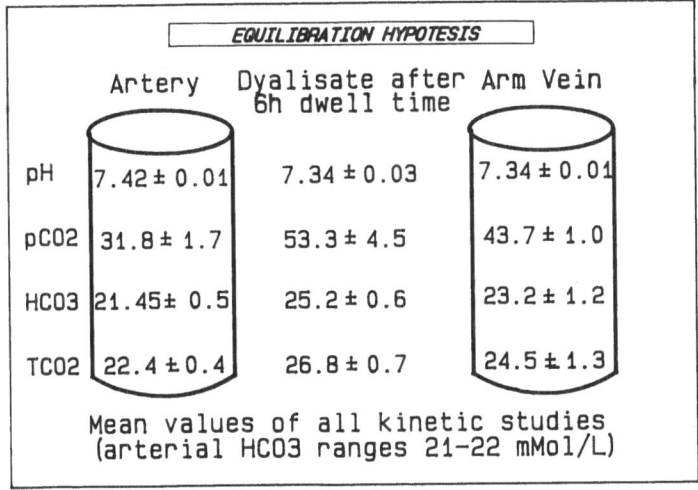

Fig. 5

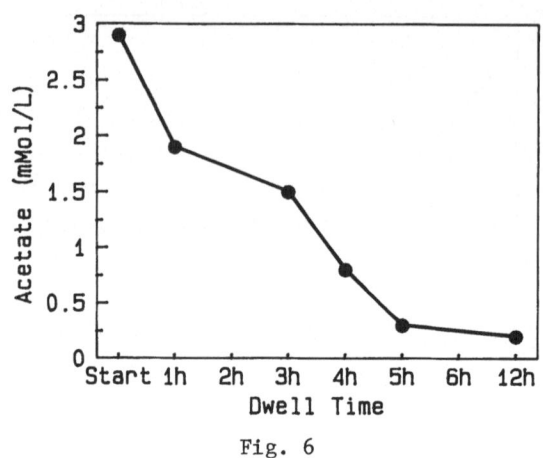

Fig. 6

quite complete after 5 hours dwell-time and at this time
almost all acetate is absorbed. This amount of alkaline
equivalent should compensate the losses of organic anions
into dialysate. At the moment there are still some problems
to solve and they mainly refer to the transfer of the clinical and experimental know-how from a laboratory status into
a routine production.

REFERENCES

1.   Boen, S.T.: In: Peritoneal Dialysis in Clinical
      Medicine, Charles C. Thomas, Springfield IL, p. 45,
      (1964).
2.   La Greca, G., Biasioli, S., Chiaramonte, S., Davi, M.,
      Fabris, A., Feriani, M., Pisani, E., Ronco, C.,
      Zen, F.: Acid-base balance on peritoneal dialysis.
      Clin. Nephrol. 16:1 (1981).
3.   Dixon, S.R., McKean, W.I., Pryor, J.E., Irvine, R.O.H.:
      Change in acid-base balance during PD with fluid con-
      taining lactate ions. Clin. Sci. 39:51 (1970).
4.   Fabris, A., Biasioli, S., Chiaramonte, S., Feriani, M.,
      Pisani, E., Ronco, C., Cantarella, G., La Greca, G.:
      Buffer metabolism in continuous ambulatory peritoneal
      dialysis: relationship with respiratory dynamics.
      Trans. ASAIO 28:270 (1982).
5.   Feriani, M., Biasioli, S., Borin, D., Brendolan, A.,
      Bragantini, L., Chiaramonte, S., Fabris, A., Ronco,
      C., La Greca, G.: Bicarbonate solutions for peritoneal
      dialysis: a reality . Int. J. Artif. Org. 8:57 (1985).
6.   Feriani, M., Biasioli, S., Borin, D., Bragantini, L.,
      Brendolan, A., Chiaramonte, S., Dell'Aquila, R.,
      Fabris, A., Ronco, C., La Greca, G: Bicarbonate buffer
      for CAPD solutions. Trans. ASAIO 31:668 (1985).

7. Feriani, M., Biasioli, S., Chiaramonte, S., Fabris, A.,
    Ronco, C., Brendolan, A., Bragantini, L., Dell'Aquila,
    R., Zambello, A., La Greca, G.: Substitution of sodium
    bicarbonate for sodium acetate/lactate in CAPD fluid.
    In: Advances in Continuous Ambulatory Peritoneal Dia-
    lysis (Kansas City) p. 16 (1986).

GLUCOSE POLYMER AS AN OSMOTIC AGENT IN CAPD

C. D. Mistry and R. Gokal

Manchester Royal Infirmary, Oxford Road
Manchester M 13 9WL England

Ultrafiltration in peritoneal dialysis is primarily an osmotically driven phenomenon achieved by means of dialysis solution made hypertonic to plasma by addition of osmotic agents. This traditional practice stemmed from early experimental work demonstrating changes in volumes of both hypo- and hypertonic solutions in the peritoneal cavity in accordance with the laws of osmosis (1,2). This seemed to confirm the "semipermeable" nature of the peritoneal membrane. Since small molecular weight solutes generate greater osmolality per unit mass, the use of crystalloids was considered as the most appropriate osmotic agents. However, amongst many of the solutes evaluated (3), only glucose proved to be safe as well as effective (4).

It was soon realised that the peritoneum was not an "ideal" semipermeable membrane but a solute permeable one, allowing rapid absorption of glucose with equally rapid dissipation of the osmotic gradient. But this was of little consequence during short dwell intermittent peritoneal dialysis (IPD). In 1976, however, the concept of long dwell equilibration peritoneal dialysis (4-10 hour dwell) (5) was introduced by Popovich and Moncrief. This led to the development of CAPD, which has revolutionised the practice of peritoneal dialysis. It is now an established alternative to haemodialysis in managing patients with end stage renal failure, but after a decade of its use several long term complications are emerging which appear to relate either directly or indirectly to the use of glucose as an osmotic agent.

GLUCOSE AND OTHER OSMOTIC AGENTS IN CAPD

Glucose, which is the only osmotic agent in common use, readily permeates through the peritoneal membrane. Using an intraperitoneal volume marker, Pyle et al.

characterised the ultrafiltration profile of glucose based
solutions (6). They demonstrated a rapid exponential
decline in the ultrafiltration rate with time in response
to a fall in osmotic gradient, due to a combination of
glucose absorption and intraperitoneal dilution. Once
equilibration of osmotic forces occured, ultrafiltration
ceased and resorption began. Since the equilibration times
was beetwen 2-3 hours with glucose solutions, the prolongation of dwell time beyond this, commonly led to reabsorption of fluid that exceeded the ultrafiltrate (negative
ultrafiltration); this was particularly noticeable in
overnight exchanges.

In addition, the continuous daily absorption of 150-
300 grams of glucose from the dialysate imposed a substantial carbohydrate load, aggravating such long term metabolic complications as hyperinsulinaemia, hyperlipidaemia
and obesity (7). More recently the prolonged exposure of
hyperosmolality and low pH of glucose have been implicated
in the insidious damage to the peritoneum and host defences
(8,9). These considerations have stimulated many investigators to search for an alternative osmotic agent with
emphasis on correcting the metabolic and ultrafiltration
deficiencies as well as achieving a more physiological
solution capable of functioning over long dwell periods.

Various osmotic agents have been tried differing
predominantly in their molecular size. Early research
workers concentrated on minimising the metabolic side
effects of glucose rather than altering the UF profile;
hence solutes of molecular size similar to or smaller than
glucose were utilised (Table 1). In the majority of cases
the rate of transperitoneal absorption exceeded the
"metabolic" capacity resulting in serious hyperosmolar
syndromes (10-13). Whilst glycerol (14-18) and amino acids
(19-22), have had some long term use, none of these have
been found suitable for general use. Large molecular weight
substances have also been tried, to modify both the UF
profile and limit metabolic side effects. Dextran (23,24)
polyanions and gelatin (25) have had limited human and
animal experimentation with disappointing results related
to relative insolubility, viscosity, allergenicity and
accumulation in the body.

The lack of success in finding a suitable alternative
agent, led to a re-examination of the fundamental role of
osmotic forces in peritoneal dialysis. In biological
systems, where water and solute requirements are similar to
those for CAPD, the osmotic effectiveness of albumin (MW
68,000) is well recognised. This physiological approach is
based on the biological model of the permeable capillary
wall, where only impermient solutes exert an osmotic force.
The osmotic flow across such membrane is determined by the
concentration gradient of impermient solutes rather than
the difference in the total number of solutes across it,
i. e. osmolality. Applying Staverman's reflection coefficient (26,27), which defines the permeability of a solute
relative to the membrane, it is possible for flow to occur
between isosmotic solutions separated by a permeable
membrane if an appropriate choice is made of solute. This
is the concept of "colloid" osmosis, with albumin as it

operates in humans as the best example. However, its use in peritoneal dialysis is limited by enormous cost.

Glucose Polymers in CAPD

Whilst none of the above substances met the needs of an ideal osmotic agent the long dwell exchange of CAPD would be best met by a large molecular weight substance. The large size would limit the rate and amount of absorption from the peritoneal cavity thus giving sustained ultrafiltration. With selection of the substance of an appropriate reflection coefficient it whould be possible to achieve UF with solutions isosmotic to uraemic plasma. Glucose polymers could subserve this role. Over the last five years we have utilised these to study the physiological concept of colloid osmosis and the role of Glucose Polymer in CAPD.

Glucose polymer is the soluble polymeric form of glucose, readily isolated by fractionation of hydrolysed corn starch. It is a mixture of oligo-polysaccharide of variable chain (dextrins) ranging from 4 to > 300 glucose units, linked predominantly by α 1-4 glucosidic and some 1-6 linkages; dextrans are similar but glucose units are linked predominantly by 1-6 linkages. GP is rapidly hydrolysed to maltose (G2) by circulating amylase (28). Maltase activity is absent in human blood but significant quantities have been demonstrated in a variety of extra intestinal tissues capable of metabolising circulating maltose (29).

Initially we studied a GP preparation with an average molecular weight 7,000 (60 % - "low MW fraction" - containing 1-12 glucose units MW 960; 33 % high MW fractions > 12 glucose units; MW 19,000) (30). Whilst effective UF was achieved its use was limited by the rapid accumulation and persistence of maltose (G2) in the blood. A second GP preparation with a molecular weight 16,800 (effectively removing the low MW fraction) was compared to standard 1.36 G solutions over 6 and 12 hour dwells (31). The results were striking; a 5 % glucose solution produced net UF greater than a 1.36 % glucose solution at both timed periods (6 hours:315 mls vs 140; 12 hours 506 vs -125; negative UF). This was in spite of the glucose polymer solution being virtually isosmotic to uraemic serum (302 vs 300 mosm/kg) throughout the 12 hour dwell, whilst the glucose solution displayed an exponential decline in the osmolality. Solute clearances were higher with GP solutions reflecting the superior UF. The percentage of carbohydrate absorbed from the peritoneal cavity was half that for G after correction for UF (at 6 hours this was 0.52 calories/ml, for glucose; 0.23 for GP). The major problem was the accumulation of maltose which rose from 0.09 mmol/1, before dialysis, to 0.79 at the end of 12 hours, the levels remaining unchanged when the dialysis was discontinued for 24 hours. During dialysis there was a peritoneal clearance of 3.5 ml/min. None of the patients observed any side effects.

The results of the studies appeared to confirm our theory of colloid osmosis as applied to glucose polymer in

Table 1

Agents	M.WT	Charge	Disadvantages
LOW MOLECULAR WEIGHT			
Glucose	182	NIL	See text
Fructose	182	NIL	Similar to glucose, hyperosmolality
Xylitol	152	NIL	Lactic acidosis hyperosmolality
Sorbitol	122	NIL	Hyperosmolality
Glycerol	92	NIL	Short UF, hyperosmolality limited to diabetics
Amino acids	75-214	-/+	No optimal formular elevated urea levels, acidosis, high costs
LARGE MOLECULAR WEIGHT			
Polyanions	90,000-500,000	-ve	Toxic to peritoneum
Polycations	40,000-60,000	+ve	Cardiovascular instability (rats)
Neutral Dextran	60,000-35,000	NIL	Low UF, absorption metabolism?
Gelatin	20,000-35,000	+/-	Allergenic, viscous accumulation/ metabolism?
Glucose Polymers	20,000-22,000	NIL	Accumulation of maltose
IDEAL OSMOTIC AGENT			
Albumin	68,000	-ve	Prohibitively expensive

CAPD with sustained UF over prolonged dwell times with isosmotic solution. If the theory was correct a hypo-osmolar solution, with the appropriate reflection coefficient would still be able to achieve positive ultrafiltration. Such was indeed the case of a 5 % GP solution (initial osmolality 277 mosm/kg) when compared to a 1.36 % glucose solution (346 mosm/kg) (32).

In order to study the effect of polymer and maltose accumulation, a 7 day study was undertaken of 7.5 % GP cycle (12 hour dwell) with 3 of 1.36 glucose (33). The results showed that a steady state level of maltose was reached by the fourth day (0.427 g/l) representing a 12 fold increase from predialysis values), without any clinical adverse effects. Over the short period the efficacy of GP was not in any doubt but longer periods of study are needed and currently we are undertaking a 3-6 months study.

CONCLUSION AND FUTURE TRENDS

Our results on GP indicate that the concept of colloid osmosis has important implications for CAPD. Firstly there is sustained Uf with an isosmolar dialysis solution which is physiological and ideally suited to long dwell dialysis. Since the phenomena also allows UF with a hypo-osmolar solution, it provides a unique opportunity to combine low and high molecular weight osmotic agents in a synergistic manner to provide a range of ultrafiltration that can be optimised for the duration of the exchange. Thus there would be a relatively larger proportion of small than large MW for short dwell exchanges, the reverse being true for long dwell dialysis. Secondly our results also indicate that colloid osmotic effect plays an important role in the reabsorption of dialysate containing crystalloids and the process may occur long before osmotic equilibration is reached, when the dialysate is relatively hypertonic to plasma and assumes greater importance with increasing dwell time. We believe that reabsorption of intra peritoneal volume involves two mechanisms, lymphatic circulation and colloid osmotic effect. Failure to take account of the osmotic effect grossly over estimates the lymphatic flow.

It is clear that for short dwell peritoneal dialysis, small molecular weight osmotic agents with rapid onset of ultrafiltration are most effective whereas the sustained action of macro molecules are more appropriate for exchanges of long duration. It seems logical that an isosmolar combination, small und large molecular weight (colloid) osmotic agents with synergetic effects of their different UF properties would be ideal for CAPD. One such possibility might be the combination of Glucose Polymer and amino acids which may improve carbohydrate and lipid metabolism as well as replacing the amino acid losses and thus maintain a positive protein balance.

As yet there is no readily available agent to replace glucose, the traditional belief that a single alternative agent to replace glucose would ideally fulfill a multitude of requirements imposed by the present CAPD system is a little naive. More recent work suggests that a "bimodal" osmotic profile containing small and large MW osmotic agents in an isosmolar concentration might be more suitable in providing a comprehensive range of ultrafiltration as well as metabolic correction and this probably represents a realistic approach toward achieving an ideal solution for CAPD.

REFERENCES

1. Wegner, G.: Chirurgische Bemerkungen über die Perito-
   nealhöhle, mit besonderer Berücksichtigung der Ovario-
   tome. Arch. Klin. Chir. 20:51 (1877).
2. Putman, J.: The living peritoneum as a dialysing membrane. Am. J. Physiol. 63:548 (1923).
3. Cunningham, R.S.: Studies on absorption from serous
   cavities III. The effect of dextrose upon the peritoneal mesothelium. Am. J. Physiol. 53:458 (1920).
4. Palmer, R.A., Quinton, W.E., Gray, J.F.: Prolonged
   peritoneal dialysis for chronic renal failure. Lancet
   1:700 (1964).
5. Popovich, R., Moncrief, J., Denchard, J., Bomar, J.B.,
   Pyle, W.K.: The defination of a novel portable/
   wearable equilibrium dialysis technique. Trans. Am.
   Soc. Artif. Int. Organs 5:64 (1976).
6. Pyle, W.K., Popovich, R.P., Moncrief, J.W.: Mass
   transfer evaluation in peritoneal dialysis. In:
   Moncrief, J.W., Popovich, R.P. eds. CAPD update.
   Masson N.Y., p. 35 (1981).
7. Hain, H., Kessel, M.: Aspect of new solutions for
   peritoneal dialysis. Nephrol. Dial. Transplant. 2:67
   (1987).
8. Duwe, A.K., Vas, S.I., Weatherhead, J.W.: Effect of
   the composition of peritoneal dialysis fluid on
   chemiluminescence , phagocytosis and bacterial activity
   in vitro. Infect. Immunity 33:130 (1981).
9. Ota, K., Mineshima, M., Watanabe, N., Naganuma, S.:
   Functional deterioration of the peritoneum: Does it
   occur in the absence of peritonitis? Nephrol. Dial.
   Transplant. 2:30 (1987).
10. Raja, R.M., Kramer, M.S., Manchanda, R., Lazaro, N.,
    Rosenbaum, J.L.: Peritoneal dialysis with fructose
    dialysate - Prevention of hyperglycemia and hyperos-
    molality. Ann. Intern. Med. 79:511 (1973).
11. Bazzato, G., Coli, U., Landinis, S., Fracasso, A.,
    Morachiello, P., Righetto, F., Scanferla, F.: Xylitol
    and low dosage of insulin: new perspectives for diabe-
    tic uraemic patients on CAPD. Perit. Dial. Bull. 2:161
    (1982).
12. Raja, R.M., Moros, J.G., Kramer, M.S., Rosenbaum,
    J.L.: Hyperosmotic coma complicating peritoneal
    dialysis with sorbitol dialysate. Ann. Intern. Med.
    73: 993 (1970).
13. Twardowski, Z.J., Khanna, R., Nolph, K.D.: Osmotic
    agents and ultrafiltration in peritoneal dialysis.
    Nephron 42:93 (1986).
14. Daniels, F.H., Leonard, E.F., Cortell, S.: Glucose and
    glycerol compared as osmotic agents for peritoneal
    dialysis. Kidney Int. 25:20 (1984).
15. Heaton, A., Ward, M.K., Johnston, D.G., Nicholson,
    D.V., Alberti, K.G.M.M., Kerr, D.N.S.: Short term
    studies on the use of glycerol as an osmotic agent for
    continuous ambulatory dialysis in end stage renal
    failure. Clin. Science 67:121 (1984).
16. Heaton, A., Ward, K.D., Johnston, D.G., Alberti,
    K.G.M.M., Kerr, D.N.S.: Evaluation of glycerol as an
    osmotic agent for continuous ambulatory peritoneal
    dialysis in end stage renal failure. Clin. Science

70:23 (1986).

17. Matthys, E., Dolkart, R., Lameire, N.: Potential hazards with the use of glycerol dialysate in diabetic CAPD patients. Perit. Dial. Bull. 7:16 (1987).

18. Matthys, E., Dolkart, R., Lameire, N.: Extended use of a glycerol containing dialysate in the treatment of diabetic CAPD patients. Perit. Dial. Bull. 7:10 (1987).

19. Oreopoulos, D.G., Crassweller, P., Kartirtzoglou, A., Ogilvie, R., Zellerman, G., Rodella, H., Vas, S.I.: Amino acids as an osmotic agent in continuous peritoneal dialysis. In: Legrain M. (ed.) Continuous Ambulatory Peritoneal Dialysis. Excerpta Medica, Amsterdam, p. 335 (1979).

20. William, P.F., Marliss, E.B., Anderson, G.H., Oren, A., Stein, A.N., Khanna, R., Pettit, J., Brandes, L., Rodella, H., Mupas, L., Dombros, N., Oreopoulos, D.G.: Amino acid absorption following intraperitoneal administration in CAPD patients. Perit. Dial. Bull. 2: 124 (1982).

21. Oren, A., Wu, G., Anderson, G.H., Marliss, E., Khanna, R., Pettit, J., Mupas, L., Rodella, H., Brandes L., Roncari, D., Kakis, G., Harrison, J., McNeill, K., Oreopoulos, D.G.: Effective use of amino acids dialysate over 4 weeks in CAPD patients. Perit. Dial. Bull. 3:66 (1983).

22. Dombros, N., Prutis, K., Tong, M., Anderson, H., Harrison, J., Sombolos, K., Digenis, G., Oreopoulos, D.G.: Six-month overnight intraperitoneal amino acid in CAPD patients: No effect on nutritional status. Nephrol. Dial. Transplant. 3:556 (1988).

23. Jirka, J., Kotkova, E.: Peritoneal dialysis by iso-oncotic dextran solution in anaesthetized dogs. Intraperitoneal fluid volumes and peritoneal concentration in the irrigation fluid. Proc. EDTA 4:141 (1967).

24. Gjessing, J.: Use of dextran as a dialysing fluid in peritoneal dialysis. Acta Med. Scand. 185:237 (1969).

25. Twardowski, Z.J., Moore, H., McGary, T., Poskuta, M., Hirszel, P., Stathakis, C.: Polymer as osmotic agents in peritoneal dialysis. Perit. Dial. Bull. 4:125 (1984).

26. Kiil, F.: Mechanisms of osmosis. Kidney Int. 21:303 (1982).

27. Herbert, S.C., Schafer, J.A., Andreoli, T.E.: Principles of membrane transport, In: Brenner, B.M., Rector FC (eds). The Kidney 2nd ed. vol I. Philadelphia, Saunders, W.B., p. 116 (1981).

28. Bibby, R.J., Davies, D., Mallick, N.P., Atherton, S.T., Wright, D.M, Rickett, R., Milner, J.: Intravenous infusion of a dextrin caloreen in human subjects: metabolic studies. Br. J. Nutr. 38:341 (1977).

29. Weser, E., Sleisenger, M.H.: Metabolism of circulating disaccharides in man and in the rat. J. Clin. Invest. 46:499 (1967).

30. Mistry, C.D., Gokal, R., Mallick, N.P.: Glucose Polymer as an osmotic agent in CAPD. In: Maher, J.F., Winchester, J.F. (eds). Frontiers in Peritoneal Dialysis. Field Rich & Assoc. New York, p. 241 (1986).

31. Mistry, C.D., Mallick, N.P., Gokal, R.: Ultrafiltration with an isosmotic solution during long peritoneal

dialysis exchanges. <u>Lancet</u> ii:178 (1987).

32. Mistry, C.D., Turner, K., Uttley, L., Gokal, R.: Can UF occur with hypoosmolar solutions across the peritoneum? <u>Perit. Dial. Bull.</u> 7: 53 (1987).

33. Mistry, C.D., Gokal, R.: The use of Glucose Polymer in CAPD: a 7 day study. <u>Perit. Dial. Bull.</u> 7:54 (1987).

EFFECTS OF LONG-TERM TREATMENT WITH HUMAN RECOMBINANT ERYTHROPOIETIN IN PATIENTS ON CAPD

Hjalmar B. Steinhauer

Department of Internal Medicine, Division of Nephrology, University of Freiburg, F.R.G.

INTRODUCTION

Anemia is a common feature in patients with chronic renal failure on regular dialysis treatment. The inappropriate low level of serum erythropoietin is known to be the major cause of anemia in these patients[1]. The development of recombinant human erythropoietin (rHuEPO) offers for the first time the possibility of an effective and continuous correction of renal anemia[2,3]. In recent publications several authors described an increase of hematocrit in patients undergoing regular hemodialysis during treatment with rHuEPO[2-7]. In the initial trials rHuEPO treatment was associated with various adverse effects such as hypertension, convulsions, fistula clotting, and increased serum creatinine, urea, and potassium [2-4].

In the present study the long-term effect of rHuEPO in patients undergoing continuous ambulatory peritoneal dialysis (CAPD) was investigated. Since rHuEPO-induced correction of anemia results in increased blood viscosity[8] and enhanced tissue oxygen supply[9] we looked into ultrafiltration and solute clearances before and under rHuEPO treatment in order to investigate the effect of increasing hematocrit due to rHuEPO therapy on dialysis efficiency in CAPD patients.

PATIENTS AND METHODS

11 clinically stable patients (female: 8, male: 3) with renal anemia (hematocrit < 28 %) undergoing CAPD took part in the study. The mean age was 42.6 years (range 26 - 65 years). One patient was anephric. The underlying renal disease was chronic glomerulonephritis in 6 patients, interstitial nephritis in 3 patients, polycystic kidney disease in 1 patient, and diabetic nephropathy in 1 patient. Informed consent was obtained from all participants prior to the trial.

RHuEPO (Cilag AG, Sulzbach/Taunus, FRG) was administered subcutaneously twice weekly in the initial dose of 50 U/kg body weight. This dose was increased for 25 U/kg body weight every 4 weeks till the target hematocrit (HKT) of 35 % had been achieved. In the event this HKT was exceeded, rHuEPO was reduced by 25 U/kg body weight.

CAPD was performed with dialysis solutions containing 1.5 % to 4.25 % glucose monohydrate (Fresenius AG, Bad Homburg, F.R.G.; Baxter, Deerfield, Ill, USA) according to the clinical requirements. Twice weekly the patients underwent a study dialysate exchange in the morning with 1.5 l, 1.5 % glucose monohydrate and a dwell time of 4 hours. These dialysates were used for the analysis of peritoneal ultra-filtration and solute clearances.

Serum electrolytes, urea, creatinine, hemoglobin, hemato-crit, platelet and white blood cell count were controlled once weekly. Serum ferritin was determined every four weeks. Clinical status and adverse effects of rHuEPO treatment were documented twice weekly. Serum and dialysate chemistry and hematological analyses were performed by routine laboratory methods. Net ultrafiltration was calculated from the diffe-rence of bag weight before infusion and after dialysis efflux. Serum ferritin was measured by enzyme-linked immuno-assay (Boehringer, Mannheim, F.R.G.).

Results are expressed as means ± SD. Statistical analysis was performed using Wilcoxon's test for combined data and linear regression analysis. The null hypothesis was rejected at $p < 0.05$.

RESULTS

During the run-in period of three months on subcutaneous rHuEPO treatment, hematocrit increased substantially in 10

Table 1. Hematological findings during rHuEPO therapy in patients undergoing CAPD

	Before rHuEPO	After rHuEPO 2 months	4 months	6 months
Transfusions (n/month)	0.13	0	0	0
Hematocrit(%)	22.9±3.1	32.1±4.2**	33.6±4.9**	31.2±5.6**
Hemoglobin (g/dl)	7.8±0.9	10.5±1.5*	9.7±2.8*	10.2±1.5*
Platelets (10^9/l)	293±113	296±94	289±78	285±70
Leukocytes (10^9/l)	5.83±1.58	5.66±1.17	5.99±1.83	6.29±1.17
Ferritin	450±596	214±347	281±347	374±353

x±SD; *p < 0.05, **p < 0.01

Table 2. Serum chemistry during rHuEPO therapy in patients undergoing CAPD

	Before rHuEPO	After rHuEPO 2 months	4 months	6 months
Sodium (mmol/l)	139±4	138±5	139±4	138±4
Potassium (mmol/l)	4.8±0.6	4.9±0.7	5.1±0.9	5.2±1.1*
Calcium (mmol/l)	2.3±o.2	2.2±0.2	2.3±0.2	2.4±0.3
Phosphate (mg/dl)	4.6±1.0	5.4±1.5	5.9±1.8*	5.3±1.6
Creatinine (mg/dl)	12.4±4.0	12.1±3.9	12.1±3.7	13.3±2.7
Urea (mg/dl)	144±40	152±44	151±46	146±44

x ± SD; *p < 0.05

out of 11 patients. Mean hematocrit rose from 22.9 ± 3.2 % to 33.3 ± 5.9 % (x ± SD, n=11) (Table 1).

In one patient, in whom the rHuEPO therapy was interrupted for 4 weeks due to an intercurrent CAPD-associated peritonitis, hematocrit rose only 4 months after the onset of rHuEPO treatment. No change of mean corpuscular volume and mean corpuscular hemoglobin concentration was observed during the study. Hematological findings before and on rHuEPO treatment are shown in table 1. Platelet number and leukocyte count as well as serum ferritin were not affected by rHuEPO. Blood transfusion rate decreased from 0.13 units per month to zero.

The mean serum levels of potassium and phosphate increased during the trial (Table 2).

No change of serum sodium, calcium, creatinine, and urea was noted. The clinical data on rHuEPO treatment are shown in table 3. Body weight, mean arterial blood pressure, heart rate, and cardiothoracic index remained unchanged during the study. Table 4 demonstrates the effect of anemia correction by rHuEPO treatment on peritoneal ultrafiltration and solute clearances. Peritoneal ultrafiltration after 4 hours dialysate dwell time (1.5 l dialysate, 1.5 % glucose monohydrate) increased from 130 ± 93 ml to 258 ± 90 ml (p < 0.05). The clearance rates of creatinine and potassium rose significantly after 6 months of rHuEPO treatment. The simultaneous increase in urea clearance lacked statistical significance.

Table 3.   Clinical data during rHuEPO in patients undergoing CAPD

	Before rHuEPO	After rHuEPO 2 months	4 months	6 months
Body weight (kg)	62.4±11.5	61.9±11.1	62.6±10.0	61.2±10.7
Mean arterial pressure (mmHg)	97±25	94±22	103±28	90±27
Heart rate (beats/min.)	80±9	82±8	81±9	80±6
Cardiothoracic index*	0.44±0.06	–	–	0.45±0.05

$x \pm SD$; *n = 6

Table 4.   Peritoneal ultrafiltration (UF) and solute clearances (Cl) during rHuEPO therapy in patients undergoing CAPD

	Before rHuEPO	After rHuEPO 2 months	4 months	6 months
UF (ml/4h dwell time)	130±93	206±117*	203±132*	258±90*
Cl urea (ml/min/1.73 m²)	5.56±0.70	6.29±1.32	6.55±1.79	6.59±1.23
Cl Creatinine 80 (ml/min/1.73 m²)	4.00±0.87	4.85±1.13	5.24±1.89	4.94±0.60*
Cl Potassium (ml/min/1.73 m²)	4.92±0.65	5.47±1.40	5.82±1.86	5.76±1.31*
Cl Phosphate (ml/min/1.73 m²)	3.49±0.62	4.12±1.01	4.62±1.25	3.59±1.05

$x \pm SD$; *$p < 0.05$

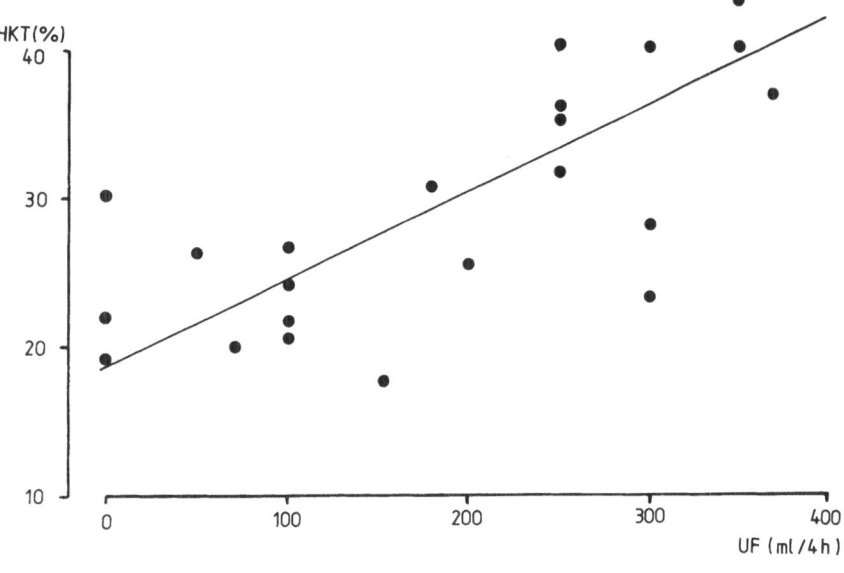

Fig. 1

The increased peritoneal ultrafiltration during rHuEPO
therapy was positively correlated with the rHuEPO-induced
rise in hematocrit (Figure 1).

Subcutaneous administration of rHuEPO was tolerated
without severe adverse effects. Five patients reported local
pain after subcutaneous injection of rHuEPO which discontinued after few minutes. Four patients required increased
antihypertensive therapy, one patient reported a flu-like
syndrome without rise in body temperature. It disappeared
within two weeks as the treatment progressed.

The mean rHuEPO dose after three months treatment was
75 U/kg body weight (range 50-100 U) twice weekly. After six
months treatment the mean rHuEPO dose was 57 U/kg body weight
(range 0-75 U).

Relationship between hematocrit (HKT) and peritoneal ultrafiltration (UF) (r = 0.6837, p < 0.001); from every
patient minimal HKT before onset of the trial and maximal HKT
on rHuEPO are shown with the corresponding UF result.

DISCUSSION

The anemia in chrònic renal failure has been postulated
to be due to a combination of absolute or relative erythropoietin deficiency[10], shortened red cell survival[11], and
inhibition of bone marrow by uremic solutes such as parathyroid hormone[12] and various polyamines[13].
Previous studies in hemodialysis patients have demonstrated

the correction of renal anemia by intravenous administration
of rHuEPO in nearly all treated patients[2-7], suggesting that
renal anemia is primarily, if not solely, due to erythropoietin deficiency[1]. In these trials the hormone was administered
intravenously three times weekly at the end of hemodialysis.
This route of administration is inconvenient for patients
undergoing CAPD. RHuEPO could be applied in CAPD patients
intraperitoneally or subcutaneously. Both routes of administration offer the purpose that the patient is able to
carry out the administration himself.

The data concerning the peritoneal absorption of rHuEPO
after intraperitoneal application are contradictory[14-16].
The mechanism by which the large molecular weight glycoprotein rHuEPO (36.000 daltons) is absorbed is not clarified.
Bargman et al.[14] described a close relationship between absorption of the hormone and dialysate absorption, indicating
a peritoneal transport by convective flux. Additionally,
peritoneal lymphatics might play an important role in the absorption of the glycoprotein[17]. The absorption of intraperitoneally applied rHuEPO was found to be 59 to 97.5 % of the
instilled amount, depending on the way of administration
together with dialysis solution or into the empty peritoneal
cavity[14]. Macdougall et al.[16] described a mean bioavailability of rHuEPO after intraperitoneal administration in CAPD
patients of only 2.9 %. According to the bioavailability data
the authors suggest that intraperitoneal rHuEPO is unlikely
to be the route of administration in CAPD patients.

Due to the lack of long-term experience with intraperitoneal administration and the observed low bioavailability of
intraperitoneally applied rHuEPO, the subcutaneous route of
administration was chosen. The dose of rHuEPO was established following the intravenous studies in hemodialysis
patients[3]. A mean of 75 U/kg body weight twice weekly induced
an increase in hematocrit from 23 % to 33 % within three
months. The adverse effects observed were necessity of
increased antihypertensive therapy in four patients, short
lasting local pain after subcutaneous injection in five
patients, and a flu-like syndrome in one patient. The
treatment had not to be discontinued in any case because of
side effects.

The hematological results of the present trial confirm
the recent findings in hemodialysis patients[3-7]. RHuEPO
treatment resulted in a partial correction of renal anemia.
The mean single dose of rHuEPO was in the same range as found
to be effective in hemodialysis patients[3]. The weekly dose
could be reduced in out trial by one third since two subcutaneous injections per week were just as effective as three
intravenous rHuEPO applications[3-6]. The observation that
less rHuEPO is necessary in CAPD patients in comparison to
patients on hemodialysis to maintain the target hematocrit of
30-35 % may be attributed to the different route of administration. A further explanation could be an improved
response to rHuEPO in CAPD patients as compared to patients
on hemodialysis.

Correction of renal anemia by rHuEPO treatment results
in a considerable improvement of physical condition and well-

being[2-4]. Despite increased appetite also observed in our patients, no gain in body weight occurred. After four months of rHuEPO therapy mean arterial blood pressure tended to increase and forced to intensify the antihypertensive treatment in four patients. After further two months the mean arterial blood pressure was below the initial value before the onset of rHuEPO treatment, indicating that hypertension in CAPD patients on rHuEPO treatment seems to be no therapeutical problem. The observed rise in serum levels of potassium and phosphate after six months of rHuEPO may depend on improved clinical condition and subsequent dietary changes as observed in hemodialysis patients [2,3]. No change of heart rate at rest and cardiothoracic index was observed after six months of rHuEPO treatment. These data confirm corresponding findings in hemodialysis patients [18,19]. By echocardiography Grützmacher et al.[18] could detect a decrease in left ventricular volume after rHuEPO-induced partial correction of renal anemia. In patients with normal contractile pattern Verbeelen et al.[19] observed a rise in stroke volume and cardiac output.

In accordance with preliminary results from our group[20], effective rHuEPO treatment resulted in an augmented peritoneal ultrafiltration. The individual analysis of hematocrit and ultrafiltration before and during the trial demonstrated that a linear, positive correlation exists between both parameters ($r = 0.6837$, $p < 0.001$). The rise in ultrafiltration also resulted in increased peritoneal clearance rates of creatinine and potassium. The change in peritoneal transport properties may be induced by increased oxygen supply of the peritoneal tissue due to higher oxygen transport capacity[21], and/or the improvement of cardiac function[18,19], indicated by the reduced left ventricular end-diastolic volume and increased cardiac output.

The present data open new perspectives in the treatment of CAPD patients. Renal anemia can be corrected by subcutaneous injection of rHuEPO. Compared to recent studies with intravenous administration of rHuEPO in hemodialysis patients, the subcutaneous rHuEPO dose per week in patients undergoing CAPD could be reduced by one third without loss of efficiency. Severe adverse effects of rHuEPO therapy did not occur. Long-term treatment with CAPD results in decreased ultrafiltration in some of the patients, probably due to peritoneal fibrosis[22,23]. The observed rise in ultrafiltration and solute clearances after rHuEPO-induced correction of anemia might improve dialysis efficiency and fluid balance especially in patients on long-term CAPD.

REFERENCES

1. Eschbach, J.W., Adamson, J.W.:Anemia of end-stage renal disease (ESRD). Kidney Int. 28:1 (1985).
2. Winearls, C.G., Oliver, D.O., Pippard, M.J., Reid, C., Downing, M.R., Cotes, P.M.: Effect of human erythropoietin derived from recombinant DNA on the anaemia of patients maintained by chronic hemodialysis. Lancet ii:1175 (1986)·
3. Eschbach, J.W., Egrie, J.C., Downing, M.R., Browne, J.K., Adamson, J.W.: Correction of the anaemia of end-stage

renal disease with recombinant human erythropoietin:
Results of the phase I and II clinical trial. New Engl.
J. Med. 316:73 (1987).

4. Bommer, J., Alexiou, C., Müller-Bühl, E., Eifert, J.,
Ritz, E.: Recombinant human erythropoietin therapy in
hemodialysis patients - dose determination and clinical
experience. Nephrol. Dial. Transplant. 2:238 (1987).

5. Casati, S., Passerini, P., Campise, M.R., Graziani, G.,
Cesana, B., Perisic, M., Ponticelli, C.: Benefits and
risks of protracted treatment with human recombinant erythropoietin in patients having haemodialysis. Br. med. J.
295:1017 (1987).

6. Bommer, J., Kugel, M., Schoeppe, W., Brunkhorst, R.,
Samtleben, W., Bramsiepe, P., Scigalla, P.: Dose-related
effects of recombinant human erythropoietin on erythropoiesis. Results of a multicenter trial in patients with
end-stage renal disease. Contr. Nephrol. Vol. 66, p 85,
Karger, Basel (1988).

7. Verbeelen, D., Hauglustaine, D., Sennesael, J.: Treatment
of the anemia of end-stage renal disease with recombinant
human erythropoietin. Neth. J. Med. 33:60 (1988).

8. Brown, C.D., Kieran, M., Zhao, Z.-H., Larson, R.H.,
Friedmann, E.A.: Treatment of azotemic, anemic patients
with recombinant human erythropoietin (rHuEPO) raises
whole blood viscosity (WB) proportional to hematocrit.
Kidney Int. 33:184 (1988).

9. Nonnast-Daniel, B., Creutzig, A., Kühn, K., Bahlmann, J.,
Reimers, E., Brunkhorst, R., Caspary, L., Koch, K.M.:
Effect of treatment with recombinant human erythropoietin
on peripheral hemodynamics and oxygenation. Contr.
Nephrol. Vol. 66, p 185, Karger, Basel (1988).

10. Gurney, C.W., Jacobson, L.O., Goldwasser, E.: The
physiologic and clinical significance of erythropoietin.
Ann. Intern. Med. 49:353 (1958).

11. Chaplin, H., Mollison, P.L.: Red cell life-span in
nephritis and hepatic cirrhosis. Clin. Sci. 12:351
(1953).

12. Meytes, D., Bogin, E., Ma, A., Dukes, P.P., Massry, S.G.:
Effect of parathyroid hormone on erythropoiesis. J. Clin.
Invest. 67:1263 (1981).

13. Radtke, H.W., Rege, A.B., LaMarche, M.B., Bartos, D.,
Campbell, R.A., Fischer, J.W.: Identification of spermine
as an inhibitor of erythropoiesis in patients with
chronic renal failure. J. Clin. Invest. 67:1623 (1981).

14. Bargmann, J.M., Breborowicz, A., Rodela, H., Sombolos,
K., Oreopoulos, D.G.: Intraperitoneal administration of
recombinant human erythropoietin in uremic animals.
Perit. Dial. Int. 8:249 (1988).

15. Boelaert, J., Schurgers, H., Matthys, E., Daneels, R.,
De Cre, M., Bogaert, M.: Recombinant human erythropoietin
pharmacokinetics in CAPD patients: Comparison of intravenous, subcutaneous and intraperitoneal routes. Nephrol.
Dial. Transplant. 3:493 (1988).

16. Macdougall, J.C., Roberts, D.E., Dharmasena, A.D., Coles,
G.A.: The pharmacokinetics of IV and IP recombinant
erythropoietin in CAPD patients. Perit. Dial. Int. 9:108
(abstract) (1989).

17. Nolph, K.D., Mactier, R., Khanna, R., Twardowski, Z.J.,
Moore, H., McGary, T.: The kinetics of ultrafiltration
during peritoneal dialysis: The role of lymphatics.

Kidney Int. 32:219 (1987).

18. Grützmacher, P., Scheuermann, E., Löw, I., Bergmann, M., Rauber, K., Baum, R., Heuser, J., Schoeppe, W.: Correction of renal anaemia by recombinant human erythropoietin: Effects on myocardial function. Contr. Nephrol. Vol. 66, p 176, Karger, Basel (1988).

19. Verbeelen, D., Bossuyt, A., Smitz, J., Herman, A., Dratwa, M., Jonckheer, M.H.: Hemodynamics of patients with renal failure treated with recombinant human erythropoietin. Clin. Nephrol. 31:6 (1989).

20. Steinhauer, H.B., Lubrich-Birkner, I., Dreyling, K.W., Hörl, W.H., Schollmeyer, P.: Increased ultrafiltration after erythropoietin-induced correction of renal anemia in patients on continuous ambulatory peritoneal dialysis. Nephron 53:87 (1989).

21. Böcker, A., Braumann, K.-M., Brunkhorst, R., Böning, D.: Effect of erythropoietin treatment on 02 affinity and performance in patients with renal anemia. Contr. Nephrol. Vol. 66, p 165, Karger, Basel (1988).

22. Slingeneyer, A., Canand, B., Mion, C.: Permanent loss of ultrafiltration capacitiy of the peritoneum in long-term peritoneal dialysis. An epidemiological study. Nephron 33:133 (1983).

23. Wideröe, T.-E., Smeby, L.C., Mjaland, S., Dahl, K., Berg, K.J., Aas, T.W.: Long-term changes of transperitoneal water transport during continuous ambulatory peritoneal dialysis. Nephron 38:238 (1984).

CONTINUOUS ARTERIO-VENOUS HEMOFILTRATION: OPTIMIZATION OF TECHNICAL PROCEDURES AND NEW DIRECTIONS

C. Ronco

Department of Nephrology, St. Bortolo Hospital
Vincenca, Italy

INTRODUCTION

In 1977 Peter Kramer treated the first patient affected by acute renal failure (ARF) with a new treatment modality called Continuous Arterio-Venous Hemofiltration (CAVH) (1).

CAVH is an extracorporeal treatment in which fluid, electrolytes and low molecular weight solutes are removed from the body by convective transport. The technique utilizes the patient's own arterial pressure to move the blood in the circuit and an ultrafiltrate with the same characteristics of those of plasma water is generated (2). The substitution of the amount of fluid lost by ultrafiltration with sterile replacement solution permits to correct electrolyte and acid base imbalances and leads to lower the patient's BUN concentration.

This simple therapy has been widely used in the recent years in the treatment of patients with severe fluid overload refractory to other therapies, patients with ARF complicated by medical or surgical problems and finally patients in which other substitutive therapies such as hemo or peritoneal dialysis were not usable due to clinical or technical problems.

While the simplicity, the easy monitoring and the good clinical tolerance were found to be the major advantages, the limits of the technique were represented by the low efficiency of the system and the extracorporeal anticoagulation (frequent clotting of the filters or patient's hemorrhagic risk).

In this paper we will try to summarize the recent improvements of the technique, the modifications in the management of the therapy and the strategies to apply in order to take the maximal advantage from the clinical use of CAVH.

VASCULAR ACCESS

The vascular access should guarantee an adequate arterio-venous gradient, it must be biocompatible, clinically well tolerated and flexible without any reduction of the inner lumen. The Scribner shunt requires surgical implantation and it partially damages the vessels of the arm making them unusable for future A-V fistulas.

On the other hand the use of large catheters enhances the risks of the arterial percutaneous cannulation and reduces the patient's clinical tolerance. In our experience the Scribner shunt should be preferred in hypotensive patient's with polytraumatisms or abdominal surgery. The cannulation of the femoral vessels should be undertaken in patients normotensive without hemorrhagic risks or other conditions which contraindicates the arterial puncture. While for the shunt a 18 G cannula is generally adequate, the choice of the catheters for the percutaneous cannulation should be made according to the patient's size, to the site of cannulation and to the extracorporeal circuit and filter available at that moment. There is no reason to use large catheters when high resistances to the blood flow are present in the extracorporeal circuit. According to that, we suggest the use of short catheters (8-10 cm long) with adequate inner diameter (2 mm) equipped with a short external segment useful to fix the catheter to the skin and to clamp the line once the vessel has been cannulated. There is a direct relationship in vitro, at a given length and diameter of the catheter, between pressures and flows through the lumen. The same relationship not always operates in vivo where the blood flows in the circuit are partially limited by the resistances of the different parts of the circuit (3). According to this observation, the maximal effort should be made to optimize the extracorporeal circuit and to reduce its overall resistance to the blood. Once this goal has been achieved the site of cannulation plays an important role (Figure 1).

1) Adequate A—V Hydrostatic Gradient
2) Low Resistance, Flexibility Safety
3) Biocompatibility, Clinical Tolerance

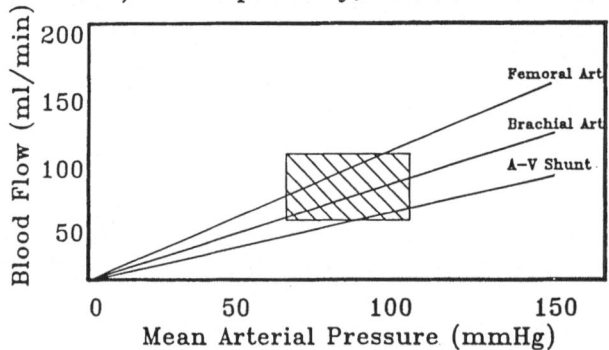

Fig. 1

Characteristics of an ideal vascular access for CAVH.
Blood flow versus mean arterial pressure in different sites of cannulation.

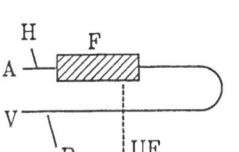

Fig. 2

Characteristics
of blood lines
for CAVH, and
different
configurations.

$$\Delta P = -\frac{8\,\eta\,l}{\pi\,r^4} - x \quad Qb$$

Requirements:
1) Adequate length
2) Adequate diameter
3) No kinking
4) Specific connections
5) Sampling ports
6) Pressure monitoring
7) Heparin and reinfusion

EXTRACORPOREAL CIRCUIT

As pointed out in several papers (4-7) various factors may influence the rate of ultrafiltration in CAVH.
Since low pressures are operating in the systems and a significant pressure drop is observed along the extracorporeal
circuit, all the skills devoted to reduce the resistance of
the circuit and to achieve its optimal performance must be
undertaken in order to increase the efficiency at the best.
Five resistances can be schematized: 1) arterial access;
2) arterial line; 3) hemofilter; 4) venous line and 5) venous access. It is evident that arterial and venous lines
should be maintained as short as possible to avoid unnecessary pressure loss along the tubes. It must be remembered
that according to the Hagen-Poiseuille law the length and
the diameter of the line are critical in conditioning the
blood flow at a given A-V pressure gradient. It is evident
that a reduction of the length of the arterial line would
permit the hydrostatic pressure of the blood to be higher
inside the filter. An asymmetric configuration of the
circuit could even be proposed keeping the arterial line
much shorter than the venous one (Figure 2). While a short
arterial line brings the filter closer to the artery, the
longer venous line can generate an higher resistance with a
consequent increase in the hydrostatic pressure inside the
filter.

HEMOFILTERS

It has been underlined that CAVH is a system operating
under conditions of low blood flow, low regiment of pressures and filtration pressure equilibrium (5-7). These observations stress the importance of adapting the size and
geometry of the hemofilter to the operational conditions. In
a standard hemofilter, as the blood passes through the
fibres, water is removed by ultrafiltration and plasma
proteins, hematocrit and viscosity increase. The consequent
decrease in hydrostatic pressure of the blood is accompanied
by an increase in oncotic pressure generated by proteins.
There may be a point inside the filter where ultrafiltration
ceases because of the equivalence between hydrostatic and
oncotic forces acting in opposite directions. In this point
the condition of filtration pressure equilibrium is achie-

ved. This condition, demonstrated by the constance of filtration fraction at different blood flows (5), generates an area of high resistance to the blood inside the filter and increases the risk of clotting in the distal region of the filter not used for filtration. The solution to this problem may consist in a modification of the blood flow geometry and resistance of the device. The possible solutions are summarized in table I. According to the Hagen-Poiseuille law a shorter filter with a larger number of fibres should permit higher blood flows at a given A-V pressure gradient and allows the filter to operate under conditions of filtration pressure disequilibrium. These considerations have led to the development of different hemofilters useful for different patients and operational conditions. AMICON has developed an entire family of hemofilters (D-10, D-20, D-30) with different surface area and geometry. While in the D-30 a standard blood path geometry, with a 0.6 sq.m. surface area can be usefully utilized for patients with stable arterial pressure and good blood flows, the shortened geometry of the D-10 with a larger cross sectional area can be very useful in patients severely hypotensive. This filter is smaller (0.20 sq.m.) but guarantees a certain amount of ultrafiltration (8-10 ml/min) in those conditions where the hypotension would preclude any other possibility of treatment (Figure 3).

Table I

HEMOFILTERS FOR CAVH

Problems:	Effects:
Low blood flows	Easy clotting
Low Pressures	Low efficiency
F.P.Equilibrium	Treatment failure

SOLUTIONS AND NEW DIRECTIONS

1) Changes in blood path geometry
2) Use of different membranes
3) Changes of the fibers' structure
4) Coating of the membrane
5) Different treatment modalities

Again, while the large hemofilter can advantageously used with a blood pump reaching ultrafiltration rates between 20 and 80 ml/min (depending on the blood flow), the short D-10 offers the maximal advantages without pumps and in severely hypotensive conditions, permitting the highest blood flow possible at a given A-V pressure gradient, because of its low resistance.

The necessity of new devices comes from the fact that since the earliest stages of CAVH, we were forced to use hemofilters which were not originally designed for spontaneous circulations but only for pumped systems. The growing interest in CAVH has stimulated the development of new products especially conceived for CAVH and arterio-venous pressure gradients. The temptative of producing a family of different hemofilters for different patients and for different conditions is the demonstration of this purpose.

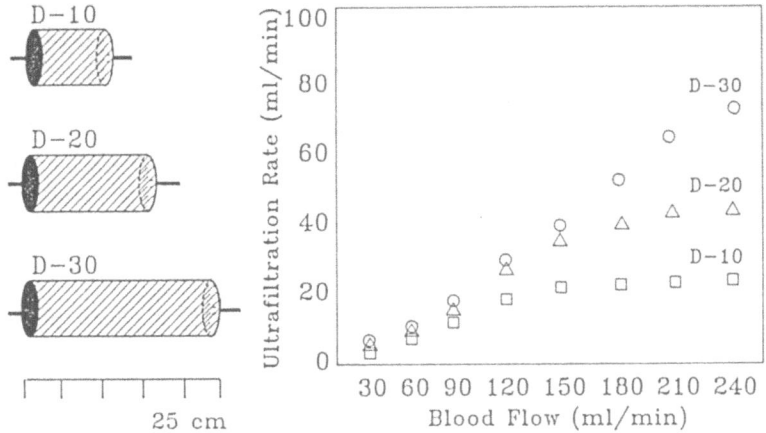

Fig. 3 Filtration versus blood flow according to filter
geometry and surface area. When a low blood flow is
present (low blood pressure, access or circuit resistance, etc.) a low resistance hemofilter should
be used obtaining the same ultrafiltration rate as
in the larger filters but having less problems of
clotting. When high blood flows can be obtained,
larger filters should be used to take the maximal
advantage from the larger surface area whom limiting
effect is demonstrated by the level of the plateau.

As reported in figure 4 new divices from different
companies have been recently proposed for CAVH with re-
markably high performances. The use of these products in
pure convective treatments, guarantee a depurative efficiency sufficient to treat even severely catabolic patients.

However other directions have been undertaken to sa-
tisfy the theoretical requirements of CAVH as a special unique procedure. One possible modification was to change the

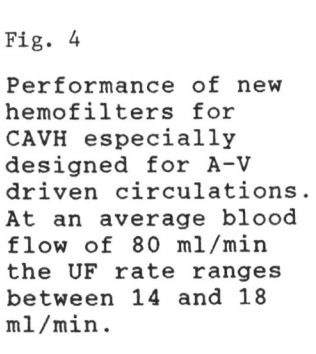

Fig. 4

Performance of new
hemofilters for
CAVH especially
designed for A-V
driven circulations.
At an average blood
flow of 80 ml/min
the UF rate ranges
between 14 and 18
ml/min.

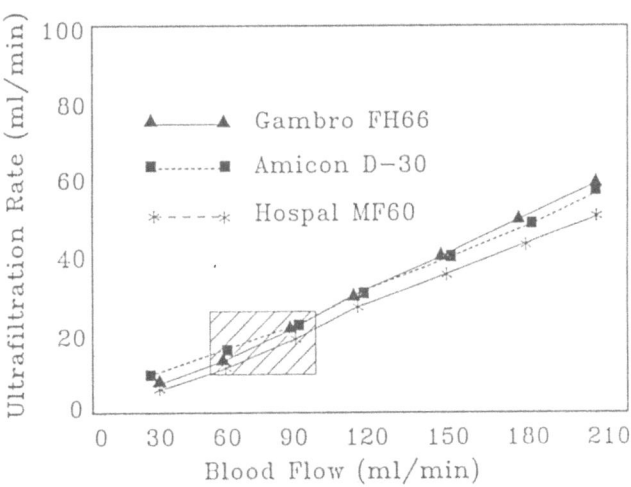

$$\Delta P = Qb \times \frac{8}{n} \frac{\eta}{\Pi} \frac{l}{r^4}$$

D-20 Device

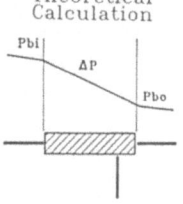

Theoretical
Calculation

Pbi

ΔP

Pbo

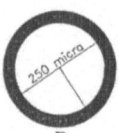

A

B

Fig. 5

Theoretical calculation
of the pressure drop in
two fibers of different
inner diameter at 100
ml/min of blood flow.

$Qb = 100$
$\eta = 3$
$l = 12.7$
$n = 5000$
$r = 100$
$\Delta P = 24.2$

$Qb = 100$
$\eta = 3$
$l = 12.7$
$n = 5000$
$r = 125$
$\Delta P = 9.8$

$$\Delta P_b = 0.4 \cdot \Delta P_a$$

structure of the hollow fiber to reduce the pressure drop according to the Hagen-Poiseuille law. Another approach consisted in the development of a new polysulphone membrane with an increased inner diameter of the fibers. The approach seems to be successfull in guaranteeing a lower resistance of the device and reducing the risk of clotting in the distal segment of the new fibers. AMICON has produced new divices (D-20 and D-30) with the new fiber. In figure 5 the rationale for the new geometry of the fibers is reported. A significant reduction of the pressure drop inside the fibers should be observed according to the Hagen-Poiseuille law. In detail, a reduction of resistance in the range of 60 % can be calculated and the first in vivo and in vitro tests confirmed this theoretical calculation. The real advantage is a greater blood flow at a given pressure with consequent increase in filtration rates and filter span life. The new filters tested in vivo presented ultrafiltration rates in the range of 10-20 ml/min and a longer span life with lower heparin requirements and constance of ultrafiltration. These points are critical in terms of treatment cost and efficiency.

As an alternative, plate devices for CAVH are also provided: despite the large housing of these hemofilters which renders them not practical at the bedside, the high biocompatibility of the polyacrylonitrile membrane and the flat sheet geometry may represent a real advantage in reducing the heparin requirement during treatment.

All these trends are useful in increasing the performances of the filters at the bedside and suggest the real necessity of new devices specific for CAVH to be available.

EFFICIENCY OF TREATMENT

In the past, several strategies have been undertaken to increase the efficiency of CAVH. The metabolic control of acute renal failure complicated or not by severe catabolism requires at least 15 liters of ultrafiltrate per day.

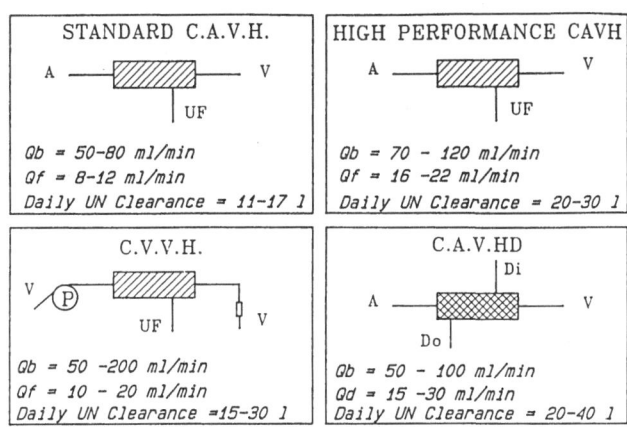

Fig. 6 Different strategies to increase CAVH efficiency.

When the classic technique couldn't achieve such a result, predilution, suction, pump assisted circulation, addition of diffusion and other techniques were used to maintain the BUN level of the patient under adequate control. CAVH is now moving towards a new era and the demonstration for that is the recent development of a series of new strategies designed to increase the efficiency of the treatment. Some of these strategies and the relevant efficiency expressed in liters/24 hours of urea clearance are summarized in figure 6. CAVH as originally conceived provides for a maximum of 17 liters/24 hours of ultrafiltrate with a pure convective transport. Pure convection is maintained with high performance CAVH but total clearance can rise up to 25 liters/24 hours. When a blood pump is utilized the blood flow can easily be increased and an overall daily clearance of 30 liters can be achieved. With the use of a blood pump, a double lumen catheter in a peripheral vein can be utilized. Finally diffusion can be added to convection by circulating dialysis fluid in the UF compartment. This can be done continuously 24 hours/day at a low speed (30 ml/min) as in continuous arteriovenous hemodialysis, or few hours/day at higher speed (100-200 ml/min) as in continuous arteriovenous hemodiafiltration. In the latter procedures a less permeable membrane can be satisfactory utilized.

Table II

AUTOMATION AND TREATMENT MONITORING

1) Roller Pump in the Arterial Line
2) Vacuum Suction in the Ultrafiltrate Line
3) Pumps or Devices for Fluid Reinfusion
4) Volume Controlled Ultrafiltration and Reinfusion
5) Dialysate Delivery System For CAVHD

CONSIDER:
-Cost Effectiveness
-Effect on Labor Intensity
-Increased Complexity

▼ ▼ ▼ ▼ ▼ ▼ ▼ ▼

NEW GENERATION OF FLUID BALANCING SYSTEMS

In conclusion, when new hemofilters providing ultrafiltration rates higher than 16-20 ml/min over a prolonged period of time are available and usable in the clinical practice, the classic limitations imposed by the low efficiency of CAVH are not any more present and alternative skills for improving the efficiency will not be necessary at all. When further efficiency is required, different alternatives are today available in the field of continuous therapies.

TREATMENT MONITORING AND AUTOMATION

Several devices and procedures have been proposed in the past to make the treatment simpler and easy to monitor. These techniques are summarized in table II. However these devices or procedures not always fulfilled the aim of semplifying the

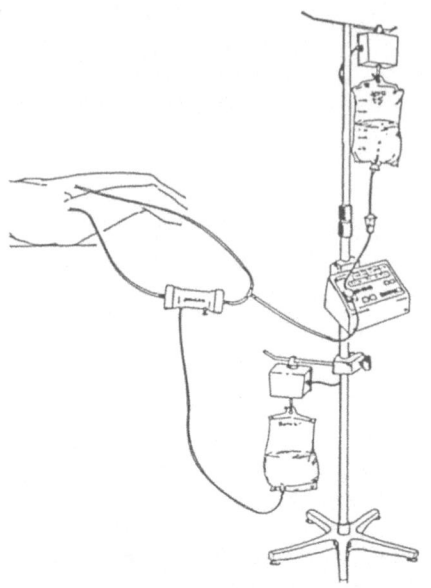

Fig. 7 Equaline Balancing System.

treatment and sometimes they even increased the labor intensity or the system complexity. For this reason a new generation of fluid balancing systems has been developed. In figure 7 we report the EQUALINE balancing system created by AMICON to monitor and control the fluid balance in patients undergoing continuous therapies. It consists on two load cells controlled by the central memory that keeps record of weight variations both of the ultrafiltrate and of the reinfusion fluid. An accurate fluid balance of the patient can be achieved and maintained for a prolonged period of time adjusting the reinfusion rate according to the recorded ultrafiltration rate and the desired weight change. The system is flexible and allows for different applications such as CAVH, CAVHD and simple infusion regulation. The system offers some advantages in terms of simplicity, it can be carried at the bedside and works just by gravity without any pump. The new generation of fluid balancing systems, may therefore contribute to improve the accuracy of treatment monitoring without increasing the complexity of the therapy.

ANTICOAGULATION

An effective anticoagulation can be achieved with a continuous heparin infusion during the treatment. The goal is the maximal anticoagulant effect inside the filter with minimal systemic effects. Several patients with high hemorrhagic risk would take advantage from an heparin free treatment or at least from a monitored administration of small amounts of heparin. The reduction of the heparin requirement during CAVH is strictly linked to specific procedures: 1) The filter must be washed before use with large quan-

Table III

ANTICOAGULATION

OBJECTIVE
To extend filter span life and performance
with minimal side effects on the patient

CONTINUOUS HEPARINIZATION

Kramer : 10 i.u./Kg/hr
Bosch et Al.:0.1−0.2 i.u./ml Qb
Ronco et Al.: 6 x Qb x (30/PTT)

ALTERNATIVES

Prostacyclin
Citrate
L.M.W. Heparin
Regional Heparinization
Predilution

IMPROVEMENT OF FILTER FLOW DYNAMICS

tities of heparinized saline to obtain the complete imbibi-
tion of the sponge-like structure of the membrane and to
get rid of all the air in the system.
2) The maximal blood flow allowed by the patient's blood
pressure must be maintained by reducing all the unnecessary resistances of the circuit. This fact ensures the
lowest filtration fraction possible at a given filtration
rate and reduces the risk of clotting.
3) The right vascular access, blood lines and filter geometry should be chosen to adapt the extracorporeal circuit
to the patient's clinical and technical requirements.
4) Use of predilution when necessary.
5) Frequent lavages of the system by flushing the filter
with saline solution.

Table III summarizes some criteria for anticoagulation
during continuous therapies. It can be noted that the first
goal is not increase of filter span life, but the best clinical tolerance to anticoagulant treatment. The formulas
reported in the table have been clinically utilized for this
purpose with satisfactory results. As an alternative, other
anticoagulant agents have been used but their use is still
under experimental research. Some substances have also been
used to coat the inner surface of the fibres in order to
make them more biocompatible. The ultimate approach in reducing the risk of clotting in the fibres is the improvement of the blood path geometry of the filter, in order to
achieve higher blood flows and lower filtration fractions at
a given arterio-venous gradient.

All the mentioned methods contribute to the reduction
of clotting problems and make the filter span life longer
even in presence of small amount of heparin or no heparin at
all.

REINFUSION OF SUBSTITUTION FLUID

The reinfusion of substitution fluids has been mostly

carried out manually in the past years. The increased understanding of CAVH and its wide use which made this procedure more familiar even in those departments where dialysis was not available, stimulated the above mentioned interest in balancing machines useful for UF and reinfusion control. These simple machines based on gravimetric control of the ultrafiltrate and a monitored feed back to the rate of reinfusion according to the desired balance do not affect the simplicity of the system and will render CAVH in the future easier and even simpler to monitor and carry out.

The quality of substitution fluid is decided upon the clinical requirements of the patient. The real improvement in recent years is represented by the use of large amounts of solutions for parenteral nutrition. An early institution of a well balanced parenteral hyperalimentation guarantees better clinical results thanks to a control of the patient's catabolism and urea nitrogen production. This leads to an improvement of the treatment efficacy because of a significantly better control of BUN levels. Other specific advantages come from the manipulation of the extracellular fluid composition made possible by CAVH treatment. Among them correction of metabolic acidosis, electrolyte derangements or abnormalities represent the most important applications for this therapy.

CLINICAL IMPLICATIONS

Once these procedures have been optimized and the performance of the treatment has been maximized for each specific patient, the clinical advantages of CAVH in the treatment of ARF become more and more evident. The critical points in the therapy of patients affected by ARF can be summarized as follows: 1) Fluid overload; 2) Accumulation of uremic toxins; 3) Electrolyte derangements and 4) Acid-base disturbances.

FLUID OVERLOAD

The operational characteristics of CAVH allow for a continuous progressive fluid removal from the patient which is generally well tolerated. Several factors have been proposed to explain the vascular stability during CAVH: the slow continuous ultrafiltration, the plasma refilling due to the isosmotic production of ultrafiltrate, the stability of the renin-angiotensin system and others . The great advantage of CAVH in our opinion depends on the possibility to dissociate the removals of sodium and water. In other words it is possible by changing the composition of the replacement solution, to remove sodium und water independently. This effect may influence the behavior of the peripheral resistances during CAVH. The hemodynamic response to fluid withdrawal by CAVH is completely different from those obtained with any other extracorporeal therapy: the stability of arterial blood pressure is in fact achieved in CAVH thanks to an inrease in cardiac index even in presence of a reduction of peripheral vascular resistances. This fact makes CAVH a first choice treatment in patients with ARF associated with myocardial disfunction and congestive heart failure and permits to achieve an improvement of the cardiac function during therapy.

SOLUTE REMOVAL

Despite its low depurative efficiency, CAVH can be successfully used as an alternative treatment in patients with ARF who cannot be treated with other therapies because of medical or technical problems. This is the case of patients with multiorgan failure, open heart surgery and other situations where hemo or peritoneal dialysis cannot be performed.

When a severe catabolic state is present several supporting procedures can be applied to improve the efficiency of the system in removing waste products:
a) The optimization of the extracorporeal circuit ensures the maximal performance of the treatment and its continuous action.
b) An adequate hyperalimentation can contribute to reduce the protein catabolic rate and its effect on BUN concentration.
c) When high blood viscosity or low blood flows are present, the use of predilution can be recommended; a consequent increase in ultrafiltration and BUN clearance (partially due to shift from RBC) can be useful to control the BUN concentrations. Furthermore the heparin requirement can be reduced.
d) Although the new generation of hemofilters allows for ultrafiltration rates ranging between 10 and 28 ml/min, sometimes the patient's hypotension does not allow for blood flows adequate to achieve the best performance of the system and the BUN level cannot be maintained under control. In these patients the efficiency of the system can be further increased by adding diffusive transport to convective one. Other strategies such as vacuum suction in the UF compartment or the use of a blood pump are still matter of discussion and they do not represent real advantages making the treatment more difficult and complicated.

CORRECTION OF ELECTROLYTE DERANGEMENTS

CAVH may be used to correct water and electrolyte imbalances by changing the composition of the substitution fluid. Hypo-hypernatremia can be corrected not only by achieving a normal plasma sodium concentration, but also by restoring the normal body sodium content. These characteristics render CAVH as particularly indicated in patients with overhydration, hyponatremia and high total body sodium. Hyerkalemia can also be corrected with CAVH: the efficiency in removing potassium is directly related to the amount of fluid removed during the treatment and its replacement with potassium free solutions. Electrolyte imbalances associated with alkalosis, where hemodialysis could worsen the clinical condition because of the large mass transfer of buffers, can also be advantageously corrected with CAVH. Calculations of ultrafiltration rate, amount and composition of the replacement solutions and blood flows may permit a theoretical prediction of the time necessary for the correction of the patient's electrolyte imbalance.

CORRECTION OF ACID-BASE DISTURBANCES

Bicarbonate loss during CAVH can easily be measured directly in the ultrafiltrate or predicted using the formula:

$$HCO3(f) = UF \times HCO3(s) \times 1.124,$$

where HCO3(f) = bicarbonate concentration in the ultrafiltrate; HCO3(s) = bicarbonate concentration in the serum; UF = total amount of ultrafiltrate, and 1.124 = average sieving coefficient for bicarbonate.

When CAVH is applied without substitution fluid in order to reduce the patient's fluid overload, bicarbonate losses are compensated by the reduction of the body volume distribution for the buffer and the serum concentration does not change significantly. On the contrary, when replacement solutions are infused to maintain the body fluid balance, the same amount of bicarbonate lost in the ultrafiltrate must be administered to achieve stable serum levels of the buffer. Finally, when CAVH is utilized to correct metabolic acidosis, the amount of HCO3 in the replacement solution must exceed the amount lost in the ultrafiltrate, providing a positive balance of the buffer.

In conclusion, when a correction of water, electrolyte or acid-base derangement is required, the rate of ultrafiltration, the rate of reinfusion, the initial plasma concentrations, the rate of metabolic production, the amount lost in the ultrafiltrate and the content of the replacement solutions, must be considered for the different solutes in order to achieve the desired final balances and plasma concentrations.

CONCLUSIONS

The use of the above mentioned procedures renders CAVH a reliable and efficient technique for the treatment of patients with ARF. Some specific advantages such as the simplicity, the easy monitoring and the easy institution make this technique a first choice treatment in several clinical conditions (Table IV). For patients with severe cardiovascular instability, multiorgan failure or polytraumatisms CAVH is infact today more than a simple alternative treatment to hemodialysis. The institution of the above described procedures and the use of new devices and materials, permit today to overcome the classic limits of CAVH such as the low depura-

Table IV

CLINICAL INDICATIONS
CAVH AS A FIRST CHOICE TREATMENT

1) Acute renal Failure with:
   - a) Cardiovascular Instability
   - b) Medical Complications
   - c) Surgical Complications

2) Multiorgan Failure

3) Non Cardiogenic Pulmonary Overhydration

4) Overhydration in Patients with:
   - a) Chronic Heart Failure
   - b) Olyguric States
   - c) Need for Hyperal
   - d) Electrolyte Imbalances
   - e) Brain Edema
   - f) Burns

5) Olyguric States in Children and Newborns

tive efficiency or the frequent clotting of the filters and will render in the near future this technique a more and more use treatment for critically ill patients.

ACKNOWLEDGEMENT

The author want to thank the friend Dr. J.P. Bosch who dedicated a lot of his precious time and competence to his understanding and knowledge in the field of CAVH.

REFERENCES

1. Kramer, B., Wigger, W., Rieger, J., Matthaei, D., Scheler, F.: Arteriovenous hemofiltration: a new simple method for treatment of overhydrated patients resistant to diuretics. Klin. Wschr. 55:1121 (1977).
2. Silverstein, M.E., Ford, C.A., Lysaght, M.T., Henderson, L.W.: Treatment of severe fluid overload by ultrafiltration. New Engl. J. Med. 291: 747 (1974).
3. Ronco, C., Brendolan, A., Bragantini, L., Chiaramonte, S., Feriani, M., Fabris, A., La Greca, G.: Continuous arterio-venous hemofiltration. Contr. Nephrol. 48:70 (1985).
4. Bartlett, R., Bosch, J.P., Paganini, E.A., Geronemus, R., Ronco, C.: Continuous arterio-venuous hemofiltration. Trans. ASAIO (1986), in press.
5. Lauer, A., Saccggi, A., Ronco, C., Belledonne, M., Glabmann, S., Bosch, J.P.: Continuous arteriovenous hemofiltration in the critically ill patient. Ann. Intern. Med. 99:455 (1983).
6. Ronco, C., Brendolan, A., Bragantini, L., Chiaramonte, S., Feriani, M., Fabris, A., La Greca, G.: Self limited dehydration during CAVH. Blood Purif. 2:88 (1984).
7. Ronco, C., Bosch, J.P., Lew, S., Fecondini, L., Brendolan, A., Bragantini, L., Chiaramonte, S., Feriani, M., Fabris, A., La Greca, G.: Technical and clinical evaluation of new hemofilter for CAVH; theoretical concepts and practical applications of a different flow geometry. In Proc. Internat. Symp. on CAVH, Vicenza 1986, Wichtig, Ed. Milano, G.La Greca, A. Fabris, C. Ronco, eds., p. 55, 1986.

IS CONTINUOUS HAEMOFILTRATION SUPERIOR TO INTERMITTENT DIALYSIS AND HAEMOFILTRATION TREATMENT?

H. G. Sieberth, H. Kierdorf

Medizinische Klinik II, RWTH Aachen
Pauwelstrasse
5100 Aachen, FRG

1. MORTALITY WITH INTERMITTENT DIALYSIS TREATMENT

An evaluation of mortality from acute renal failure
(ARF) over the period from 1951 to 1985 reveals a rise in
average mortality from about 30 % in 1951 to roughly 70 % in
1985 (Fig. 1). These figures are drawn from 212 references
in the literature assigned to the date of publication or the
date at which the publication was received, even where
treatment had taken place earlier. Two causes are generally
cited for this rise.

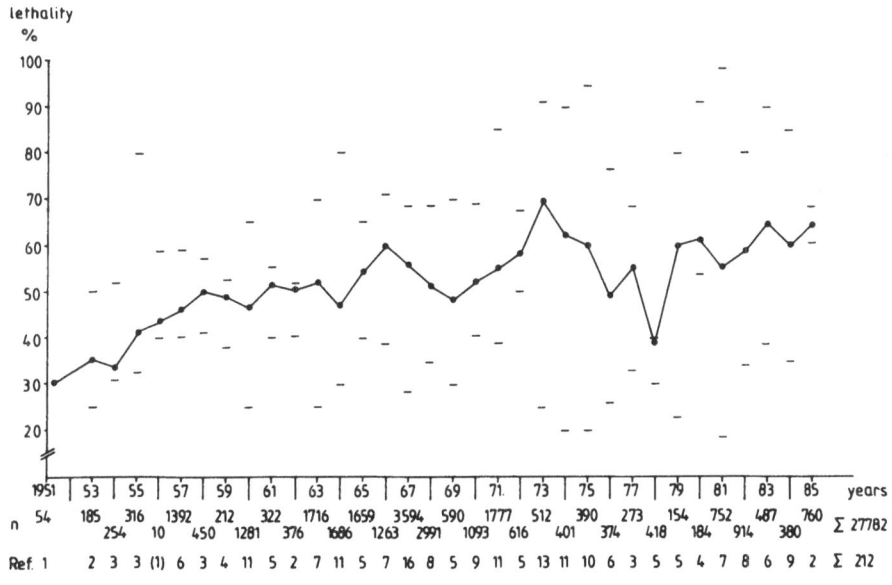

Fig. 1   Evaluation of mortality from acute renal failure
from 1951 to 1985 drawn from 212 references.

1. There has been a substantial improvement in shock prophylaxis, leading to a reduction in the number of uncomplicated acute renal failure.

2. Owing to improvements in intensive care, acute renal failure now affects many patients who would formerly have died before the condition could occur.

In our own group of cases, there was a mortality of 67.9 % for 980 patients with acute kidney failure, who also received dialysis. The average age was 49 years, with a male/female ratio of 1.7:1. These statistics include acute kidney failure patients from the Cologne University Clinic over the period from 1966 to 1981.

It is noticeable that the mortality for patients treated primarily in an intensive care unit between 1966 and 1985 remained virtually constant (Fig. 2).

It would therefore be possible to argue that the rise in mortality paralleled the creation of intensive care units. Where intensive care units with a high concentration of severe cases already existed, mortality remained roughly the same, at 70 %.

Analysis of cases according to the number of vital function disturbances occurring in addition to acute renal failure reveals a rise in mortality from 12 % with no additional vital function disturbances to 96 % when four vital functions are disturbed (Table 1).

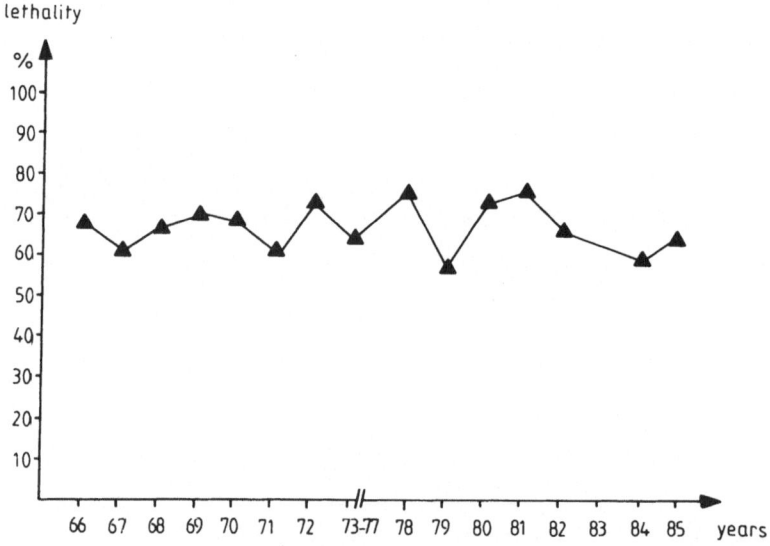

Fig. 2   Mortality of primarily intensive care-treated ARF
patients between 1966 and 1985.

Table 1. Relationship between vital function disorder
and lethality in dialysis patients
with acute renal failure (ARF)

vital function disorder	dialysis patients with ARF	lethality	%
0	101	12	12
1	269	148	55
2	272	217	80
3	164	147	89
4	55	53	96
	861*	577*	67**

* total
** mean

In this context, it is important to note that a similar
increase in mortality was found for patients with several
vital function disturbances without acute kidney failure[8].
This poses the question of whether mortality in cases of
acute renal failure is determined solely by the number and
severity of vital function distubances, irrespective of
dialysis treatment, and whether further optimization of
kidney replacement therapy can achieve any substantial
reduction in mortality.

A comparison of the number of vital function disturbances before and during dialysis treatment of 243 patients
with acute renal failure showed that the number of vital
function disturbances increased considerably during dialysis
therapy (Table 2). Here again, it is necessary to ask
whether an improvement of intensive care measures, and
particularly of kidney substitution therapy, enables us to
prevent an increase or even bring about a reduction in the
number of vital function disturbances during dialysis
treatment.

Table 2. Progression of vital function disorder during
intermittend dialysis treatment

vital function disorder	before dialysis treatment	during dialysis treatment
0	69	26
1	102	44
2	50	86
3	19	69
4	3	18
	243	243

2. FORMS OF INTERMITTENT DIALYSIS AND HAEMOFILTRATION TREATMENT

In dialysis, substances diffuse from the blood to the haemodialysis solution in accordance with the concentration gradient. In Fick's principle, the diffusion rate is dependent on molecular size. In haemofiltration, by contrast, elimination takes place by convection. All substances dissolved in the plasma water are eliminated with equal effectiveness up to a maximum molecule size. The cut-off point for maximum molecule size is determined by the pore size of the membrane. Comparing the two methods, this implies that low-molecular-weight substances will be eliminated more effectively by haemodialysis and high-molecular-weight substances by haemofiltration. The elimination rate per unit time for a particular substance is naturally fixed via the dialysance for filtrate volume. The total quantity of a substance eliminated is also dependent on plasma concentration and length of treatment. In the continuous arteriovenous haemofiltration method introduced by Kramer et al. in 1977[14], the motive force was arterial blood pressure. The filtrate volume was dependent on blood pressure and the capacity of the selected filter. The advantage of the technique was its ease of handling. Monitoring devices, in particular an air trap, were not required. Its disadvantage was that an artery had to be tapped and that the filtrate volume could not be determined in advance.

Continuous venovenous haemofiltration requires a blood pump with air trap and automatic tube clamps. Modern haemofilters are, however, capable of achieving any reasonable desired filtrate volume with venovenous filtration.

The most important problem associated with long-term filtration is that of fluid balance. Slight errors in the balance may cumulate over a longer period, leading to substantial balance errors entailing patient risk. For this reason, haemofiltration should nowadays as far as possible be performed only with automatic fluid balancing equipment, which safeguards against such errors.

Today there is a choice of electrical and mechanical balancing devices[18]. An electronic balancing device developed in this clinic obtains a zero balance, i. e. the device is designed to equalize the supplied and filtered volumes. A negative balance is obtained by pumping the desired volume from the receiving reservoir via an additional tube pump. A correspondingly lower volume of substitution solution is returned to the patient via the zero-balanced device. Even with poor pressure values, filtrate volumes of 20 to 30 l are easily achieved with continuous haemofiltration, without affecting circulation.

We prefer to carry out continuous haemofiltration at a high blood flow rate. If the filtrate flow rate becomes excessive, a restricting clamp or, more elegantly, a calibrated tube pump, is used to set the required flow.

A high blood flow rate reduces the risk of coagulation in the system. Filter flow times under these conditions were

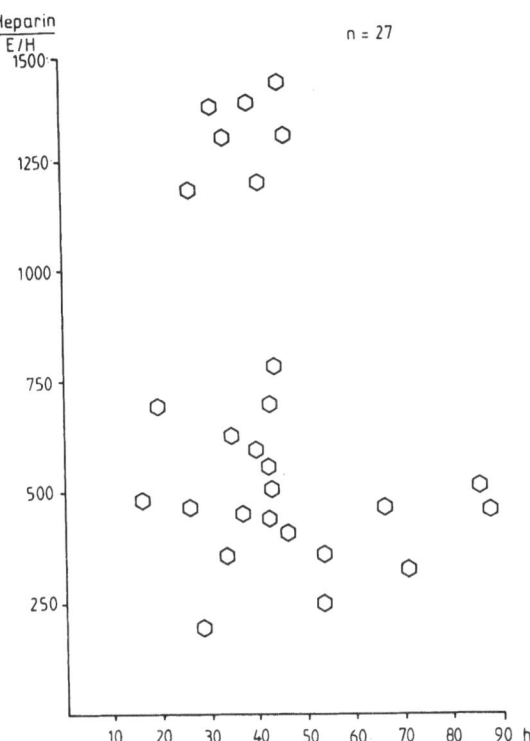

Fig. 3 Relationship between heparin and filter flow times
at high blood flow rates

roughly equal for high and low heparin volumes (Fig. 3). We
now use approximately 500 U heparin per hour.

With somewhat greater technical effort, it is also
possible to perform continuous haemodialysis or haemodiafil-
tration[20]. We do not use this technique, as we see no
advantages as compared to continuous haemofiltration at high
filtrate volumes.

3. ADVANTAGES AND DISADVANTAGES OF INTERMITTENT AND CONTINUOUS TREATMENT

Further it will be considered from a theoretical
viewpoint whether continuous kidney substitution therapy,
i. e. continuous haemofiltration (CH) is better adapted to
physiological conditions than intermittent treatment, and
thus of greater potential benefit. Currently available
clinical data will then be discussed.

The fluctuations in retention values, electrolytes and
body fluid content encountered even with daily intermittent

treatment can be eliminated completely by continuous haemo-filtration. Unlike arteriovenous haemofiltration, venovenous haemofiltration at filtrate volumes in excess of 20 l per day invariably results in a decrease in retention values. The additional haemodialysis or haemofiltration frequently required with continuous arteriovenous haemofiltration are unnecessary. Fluctuations in the plasma sodium concentration and varying hydration states result in substantial fluid shifts via the haemato-encephalic barrier, with consecutive cerebral oedema[12]. These changes are tolerated very poorly, especially by older patients and those with arteriosclerotic cerebral affections. Clinically, it is our impression that patients treated by continuous haemodialysis exhibit fewer cerebral complications, and that transit syndromes in particular are less frequent and less pronounced.

Especially with oligo-anuric patients, hyperhydration frequently occurs during intermittent treatment, due to parenteral feeding and drug infusions between dialyses. Fluid infiltration to the lungs in cases of shock lung and pneumonia is particularly dangerous. This infavourable situation, almost invariably associated with deterioration of the blood gases, can be avoided by continuous haemofiltration.

In patients with a weak circulatory system, the fluid balance can be optimized with the aid of a Swan-Gantz catheter to obtain the most favourable cardiac output according to Starling's curve. This is of particular importance with patients requiring catecholamines and patients with intra-aortal balloon pulsation.

Continuous haemofiltration also has significant advantages for parenteral feeding. Oligo-anuric patients frequently need infusion of high-osmolality solutions. This requirement is obviated under continuous haemofiltration, since any desired fluid volume can be given for parenteral feeding or administation of drugs. A corresponding volume of fluid is then simply removed from the filtrate reservoir for negative balancing.

The nitrogen balance for continuous haemofiltration patients is easily determined. Manufacturers detail nitrogen inputs on their infusion solutions. The nitrogen content in the filtrate and excreted urine are easy to determine[10]. Nitrogen balances for intermittently haemodialysed patients can be determined only with greater effort and a greater margin of error.

Drug dosing is also easier to manage with continuous haemofiltration. Doses of drugs which can be eliminated by continuous haemofiltration are simpler to calculate. For a rough approximation, the filtrate volume and the remaining renal clearance can be added to give the total clearance. Using this value, dose and dose interval can then be read off from the dosage tables for patients with renal insufficiency[19]. This does not, of course, apply to substances which are largely tubularly secreted, e. g. penicillin.

	Glomerular Filtrate	Haemofiltrate
	25 ml/min	25 ml/min
Digoxin clearance	25 ml/min	25 ml/min
Penicillin clearance	100 ml/min	25 ml/min

Patients with acute renal failure receiving intermittent dialysis or haemofiltration treatment frequently tend to hypophosphataemias, requiring phosphorus substitution. Hypophosphataemias of this kind can be avoided in continuous haemofiltration by adding the required quantity of phosphorus to the substituted fluid. We routinely use a concentration of 1.5 mmol/l of phosphate.

A previous disadvantage of continuous haemofiltration was that patients with severe lactate acidosis received substitution solutions containing lactate. In the last few months, it has become possible to use commercially available bicarbonate solutions. The bicarbonate is added to the substitution fluid shortly before use. The selected method excludes bacterial contamination.

Puncturing of the arteria femoralis is a risk associated with continuous arteriovenous haemofiltration. Puncture involves a danger of arterial bleeding and arterial thrombosis. This bleeding risk is considerably reduced in venovenous haemofiltration.

The lack of opportunity for patient mobilization is often seen as a further disadvantage of continuous haemofiltration. We therefore use continuous haemofiltration with severely ill patients who are in any case immobilized. In venovenous as opposed to arteriovenous haemofiltration, therapeutic measures are much less seriously restricted. If the patient's condition improves to a point at which he can again be mobilized, venovenous haemofiltration is no longer necessary and intermittent treatment may be resumed.

The most significant and perhaps the only really important disadvantage of continuous haemofiltration is the need for continuous heparinization, currently ruling out use of CH in bleeding patients or haemophilia risk groups. Continuous use of prostacyclin analogues has not yet been sufficiently researched and therefore not (yet) be recommended.

Apart from the important practical advantages of this form of treatment, certain other, still theoretical, considerations should be noted.

In haemodialysis, a fall in the leucocyte and thrombocyte counts to as little as 50 % of the original value is frequently observed, depending on the membrane used[9]. With sequestration of the leucocytes in the lung capillaries, a drop in the PO_2 concentration has also been observed[1]. The probable cause is complement activation at the membrane[2,9]. These changes have so far been observed neither in continuous nor in intermittent haemofiltration[1,4].

From studies to date, it may be assumed that low-molecular-weight proteases and their biologically active fission products are responsible for the hypercatabolism noted at the onset of acute renal failure[6,7,21]. The filtrates of patients with acute uraemia exhibit high proteolytic activities, whereas no such activity is detected in the ultrafiltrates of patients with normal function. High proteolytic activities have been demonstrated both in the filtrate and in the urine of patients with multi-organ failure, especially those with simultaneous sepsis[21]. It has not yet been possible to determine whether continuous elimination of the proteases has a favourable effect on the course of acute renal failure.

4. RESULTS OF CONTINUOUS HAEMOFILTRATION TREATMENT

Results of continuous haemofiltration treatment are cited by various authors[3,15,16]. Almost all authors report favourable results, only Kohen et al.[13] describing a negative influence of CH in three cases. The analyses are, however, retrospective, with a small number of cases, producing no significant results.

Evaluation of our first 79 continuous haemofiltration patients shows a mortality distinctly lower than for our dialysis patients, at 54 % as opposed to 68 % (n = 980).

Another surprising result showed that the filtrate volume per day was higher for the surviving patients than for those who died (Table 3). There were no differences in retention values and age. There were, however, more men than women in the group who died. The significance of these results offers much scope for speculation. Certain is only that higher filtrate volumes enable retention values to be reduced to a more favourable range.

Table 3. Clinical data of ARF patients treated with CH

	survivers n = 11	death rate n = 16
filtrate l/day	17.8±4.9	10.7±7.2 < 0.01
urea (mmol/l) before treatment	43.4±10.5	32.1±11.7
creatinine (µmol/l) before treatment	466±123	348±114
♂ : ♀	5:6	13:3
age X years	55.4	56.3
days of treatment	17.5±8.7	8.8±6.3

In recent years, we have used continuous haemofiltration particularly for patients whose prognosis was regarded
as especially unfavourable. Results for 1985 to 1987 may be
presented here. Over this period, a total of 259 patients
with acute renal failure were treated by dialysis and
haemofiltration. For 63 patients treated in 1985 the
mortality was 67 %, for 94 patients in 1986 65 % and for
102 dialysis patients in 1987 62 %. As compared to the
overall mortality referred to above, these figures lie below
the average for purely intermittent dialysis treatment. A
comparison between intermittently and continuously treated
patients reveals a different picture, however. In 1985, the
mortality for continuously treated was even lower than for
intermittently treated patients. In the following years,
there was a substantial fall in the mortality for intermittently treated patients, while the mortality for continuously treated patients in 1987 was even 30 % higher than
for intermittently treated patients. As already noted, total
mortality in 1987 was nonetheless at its lowest, with 62 %
(Table 4).

Table 4. Mortality of ARF patients treated by
intermittend haemodialysis or CH

	intermittend treatment			continuous treatment			both treatments		
	n	+	%	n	+	%	n	+	%
1985	38	27	(71)	25	15	(60)	63	42	(67)
1986	66	39	(59)	28	22	(79)	94	61	(65)
1987	59	29	(49)	43	34	(79)	102	63	(62)
	163	95	(58)	96	71	(73)	259	166	(64)

We interpret the fall in total mortality for patients
with acute renal failure, the low mortality for the intermittently treated and the high mortality for the continuously treated patients as follows. Continuous haemofiltration was considered to be indicated particularly for
patients whose prognosis was seen as infavourable. Given a
reduction in total mortality, it could then be argued,
naturally with all due caution, that despite the higher
mortality in this group, the prognosis of the unfavourable
cases was nonetheless improved as a result of continuous
dialysis treatment.

Mathematical proof of this thesis can, of course, be
provided only by a controlled study.

5.   INDICATIONS AND CONTRA-INDICATIONS FOR CONTINUOUS
HAEMOFILTRATION

On the basis of our experience to date, we regard
continuous haemofiltration as indicated mainly in cases of

Table 5.   Indications and contra-indications for CH in cases
of severe vital function disorder

Indications	Contra-Indications
1. shock	massive bleeding
2. acute respirat. distress syndrome (ARDS)	
3. cardiac insufficiency	
4. multi organ insufficiency	
5. unconsciousness	

severe vital function disturbance (Table 5). We see only
severe bleeding or substantial risk of bleeding as a
contra-indication for continuous haemofiltration.

SUMMARY

1.   Mortality in cases of acute renal failure has in-
       creased from roughly 30 % to roughly 70 % in recent
       decades.

2.   The rise paralleled the creation of intensive care
       units. In such units, more seriously ill patients
       reach the stage of acute renal failure. Before the
       advent of intensive care units, these patients died
       before acute renal failure could occur.

3.   From a theoretical viewpoint, continuous haemofiltra-
       tion (CH) has substantial advantages as opposed to
       intermittent dialysis and haemofiltration treatment.

4.   No clinical proof of the superiority of continuous
       haemofiltration to the intermittent techniques has yet
       been provided.

5.   In our own patient group, total mortality for acute
       renal failure patients decreased following adoption of
       continuous haemofiltration. During a selected period
       of use of continuous haemofiltration for patients with
       an unfavourable prognosis, however, the mortality with
       continuous haemofiltration was higher than that with
       the intermittent methods.

REFERENCES

1.   Böhler, J., Kramer, P., Gölke, O: Leukocyte counts
       and complement activation during pumpdriven and
       arteriovenuoushemofiltration. Contrib. Nephrol. 36:15

arteriovenuoushemofiltration. <u>Contrib.</u> <u>Nephrol.</u> 36:15 (1983).

2. Craddock, P.R., Fehr, J., Brigham, K.L., Kranenberg, R.S., Jakob, H.S: Complement and leukocyte mediated pulmonary dysfunction in hemodialysis. <u>New</u> <u>Engl.</u> <u>J.</u> <u>Med.</u> 296:760 (1977).

3. Dodd, N.J., O'Donovan, R.M., Bennett-Jones, D.N., Rylance, P.B., Bewick, M., Parsch, V., Weston, M.J.: Arteriovenuous hemofiltration: A recent advance in the management of acute renal failure. <u>Brit.</u> <u>Med.</u> <u>J.</u> 287:1008 (1983).

4. Colper, T.A.: Continuous arteriovenuous hemofiltration in acute renal failure. <u>Am.</u> <u>J.</u> <u>Kidney</u> <u>Dis.</u> 6:373 (1985).

5. Grittmann, G.: Akutes Nierenversagen bei Patienten des Aachener Klinkums von 1984 bis 1985, Prognose, Verlauf und Nachuntersuchung. Dissertationsschrift, Med. Fak. der RWTH Aachen (1987).

6. Hörl, W.H., Heidland, A.: Enhanced proteolytic activity-cause of protein catabolism in acute renal failure. <u>Am.</u> <u>J.</u> <u>Clin.</u> <u>Nutr.</u> 33:1423 (1980).

7. Hörl, W.H., Stepinski, H., Schäfer, R.M., Wanner, C., Heidland, A.: Role of protease in hypercatabolic patients with renal failure. <u>Kidney</u> <u>Int.</u> 24 (Suppl. 16): S-37 (1983).

8. Imig, H., Schütt, A.: Die Prognose der Kranken auf einer chirurgischen Intensivstation. <u>In:</u> Sieberth, H.G. (Hrsg.) Akutes Nierenversagen, Verlag G. Thieme, Stuttgart - New York, S. 114 (1979).

9. Jakob, A.I., Gravellas, G., Zarco, R.: Leukopenia, hypoxia and complement function with different hemodialysis membranes. <u>Kidney</u> <u>Int.</u> 18:505 (1980).

10. Kierdorf, H., Kindler, J., Sieberth, H.G.: Nitrogen balance in patients with acute renal failure treated by continuous arteriovenous hemofiltration. <u>Nephrol.</u> <u>Dial.</u> <u>Transplant.</u> 1:72 (1986).

11. Kindler, J., Frisch, J., Meister, M., Grittmann, G., Jenn, I., Sieberth, H.G.: Akutes Nierenversagen beim Multiorganversagen. <u>Intensivmed.</u> 23:214 (1986).

12. Kleemann, C.R.: CNS Manifestation of Disordered Salt and Water Balance. <u>Hospital</u> <u>Practice</u> <u>Mag.</u> p. 59 (1979).

13. Kohen, J.A., Whitley, K.Y., Kjellstrand, C.M.: Continuous arteriovenous hemofiltration: A comparison with hemodialysis in acute renal failure. <u>Trans.</u> <u>Am.</u> <u>Soc.</u> <u>Artif.</u> <u>Intern.</u> <u>Org.</u> 31:169 (1985).

14. Kramer, P., Wigger, W., Rieger, J., Matthaei, D., Schieler, F.: Arteriovenous hemofiltration: A new and simple method for treatment of overhydrated patients resistant to diuretics. <u>Klin.</u> <u>Wschr.</u> 55:1121 (1977).

15. Mauritz, W., Sporn, P., Schindler, I., Zadrobilek, E., Roth, E., Appel, W.: Akutes Nierenversagen bei abdomineller Sepsis. Vergleich von Hämodialyse und kontinuierlicher arteriovenöser Hämofiltration. <u>Anästh.</u> <u>Intensivther.</u> <u>Notfallmed.</u> 21:212 (1986).

16. Paganini, E.P., O'Hara, P., Nakamoto, S.: Slow continuous ultrafiltration in hemodialysis resistent oliguric acute renal failure patients. <u>Trans.</u> <u>Am.</u> <u>Soc.</u> <u>Artif.</u> <u>Intern.</u> <u>Org.</u> 3:173 (1984).

17. Schultheis, R., Brings, W., Glöckner, W.M., Sieberth,

H.G.: Device for Controlled Cyclic Substitution during Spontaneous Filtration. In: Sieberth, H.G., Mann, H. (Hrsg.) Continuous Arteriovenous Hemofiltration (CAVH). Verlag Karger, Basel - München, p. 64 (1985).

18. Schurek, H.J., Biela, J.D.: Further Improvement of a Mechanical Divice for Automatic Fluid Balance in CAVH. In: Sieberth, H.G., Mann, H. (Hrsg.) Continuous Arteriovenous Hemofiltration (CAVH). Verlag Karger, Basel - München, p. 79 (1985).

19. Sieberth, H.G.: Dosierung von Pharmaka und Auswahl der Substitutionslösung unter kontinuierlicher Hämofiltration. In: Intensivmedizin 1987 (VIII. Int. Symp. über Probleme der Notfallmedizin und Intensivtherapie, 21.-23. Mai 1987, Verlag G. Thieme, Stuttgart - New York, S. 79 (1987).

20. Siegler, M.H., Teehan, B.P., Valkenburg, van D.: Solute treatment in continuous hemodialysis: A new modality for treatment of acute renal failure. Kidney Int. 32:562 (1987).

21. Wanner, C., Schollmeyer, P., Hörl, W.H.: Urinary proteinase activity in patients with multiple traumatic injuries, sepsis, or acute renal failure. J. Lab. Clin. Med. 108:224 (1986).

THERAPEUTIC APHERESIS UPDATE

Hans J. Gurland

Nephrology Department, University Hospital Munich
Grosshadern, P.O. Box 701260, D-8000 Munich 70, FRG

The fact that the father of both hemodialysis [1] and plasmapheresis [2] is one and the same, and that he proposed both forms of therapy in the same year, provides an historical link between the two modes of treatment. The advent of on line centrifugation systems for apheresis in the mid-fifties, however, moved this new technique into the domain of hematologists. Plasma donation procedures have improved immensely in recent years. They are usually performed by blood banks and as such will not be considered here. This survey will deal only with therapeutic apheresis, which nowadays is practiced both by hematologists and nephrologists, and has become an integral part of the training programs in both disciplines.

The take-home message from this article is very simple: "In the field of apheresis, technical progress outpaces the clarity of indications." Accordingly, emphasis shall be placed not only on the approved indications and ongoing trials, but also on newer technical developments now in use and those projected for the future. Consensus indications for apheresis have been published by the scientific bodies of several associations [3,4,5]. These describe up to 20 diseases for which apheresis is considered standard therapy. Results from controlled trials and enhanced levels of practical experience have, however, changed the picture somewhat.

In the United States, private or governmental insurances will only reimburse therapies which have been demonstrated to be safe and effective. The current list of diseases "reimbursable" under Medicare is surprisingly broad:
- plasmapheresis for myasthenia gravis (acute intervention),
- plasmapheresis for Goodpasture's syndrome,
- plasmapheresis for Guillain Barré syndrome,
- plasmapheresis for macroglobulinemia,
- plasmapheresis for hyperglobulinemia,
- leukapheresis for leukemia,
- plasmapheresis over charcoal for pruritus in cholostatic liver disease,
- plasmapheresis for thrombotic thrombocytopenic purpura (TTP),
- plasmapheresis for chronic inflammatory demyelinating polyneuropathy (CIPD),
- plasmapheresis for deteriorating life-threatening rheumatoid vasculitis, and
- plasmapheresis for deteriorating life-threatening lupus erythematosus (LE).

From various reports presented at the 2nd International Congress of the World Apheresis Association held in Ottawa from May 18-20, 1988 it would appear that the following diseases should be added to the list of re-imbursable indications:
- hypercholesterolemia treated with adsorption or precipitation techniques,
- pemphigus,
- coagulation factor inhibitors,
- Grave's opthalmopathy,
- Refsum's disease, and
- certain classes of drug overdose and poisoning.

As space is limited, only a few but important indications shall be high-lighted in the following.

Multiple sclerosis (MS) is of special interest because of its annual in-cidence of approximately 500 cases per million. Several clinical trials have been or are presently being performed.
- The Canadian Apheresis Study Group has enrolled 136 patients to date; 200 are required [6].
- Dau in Evanston, Illinois has randomly treated 116 MS patients in 59 true and 57 sham situations [7].
- Schmitt in Rostock, GDR is presently comparing plasma exchange with immuno adsorption in a three-arm study [8]; and
- Khatri in Milwaukee, Wisconsin has completed a double blind controlled study and is now treating 200 patients in an open fashion with weekly plasma exchanges [9].

The results of these activities provide a growing body of data in support of the benefit of plasma exchange in conjunction with immunosuppressive therapy in the treatment of MS. However, definitive judgement must await the completion of the ongoing trials.

Many advocates of apheresis believe that there has been a gradual im-provement in the results of treatment in rapidly progressive glomerulonephritis (RPGN) with the empirical and polypragmatic use of immunosuppressive drugs and plasma exchange. The broad therapeutic strategy is to firmly diag-nose the disease etiology, to employ apheresis to rapidly decrease the level of circulating autoantibodies, then to employ immunosuppression to prevent their reoccurence.

Lockwood and his group at Cambridge have developed assays to detect the presence of circulating antiglomerular basement membrane antibodies in Goodpasture's syndrome and antineutrophil cytoplasm autoantibodies in systemic vasculitis, especially Wegener's granulomatosis and microscopic polyarteritis. Detection and discrimination of such antibodies enables rapid diagnosis and early treatment. In recent work [10], the Cambridge group was able to show that the incidence of antiglomerular basement membrane antibody and antineutrophil cytoplasm autoantibody in RPGN occurs in a ratio of 1:6. This ratio is similar to that seen in the comparison of linear to non-linear deposits in renal biopsies from patients with RPGN, suggesting that the indication for apheresis in this group of renal disorders may be soon expanded to include patients with non-linear glomerular deposits. After having seen satisfactory recovery of renal function in dialysis-dependent patients with both antiglomerular basement and antineutrophil cytoplasm autoantibody positivity, Lockwood now recommends plasmapheresis for such patients, even though they might already be on dialysis.

Systemic lupus remains one of the most controversial indications for apheresis therapy. The lack of double-blind controlled studies is not for want of trying. Rather it stems mainly from the extreme heterogeneity of the syndrome and the resultant difficulty in assembling groups of patients with lupus who are sufficiently similar so that adequate controlled studies may be conducted. Also, controlled studies in patients with life-threatening diseases pose a variety of ethical problems.

One controlled trial of plasmapheresis in 86 patients as adjunct to conventional therapy in severe lupus nephritis was carried out by the Lupus Nephritis Collaborative Study group, headed by Lewis [11]. The recently published outcome showed a mean follow-up period of 13 months comparing plasma exchange and control groups. There was no significant difference in any evaluated outcome parameter.

Moreover, both Austin in 1985 [12] and McCune in 1988 [13] showed favourable results in the treatment of severe lupus nephritis with intravenous cyclophosphamide prompting many to abandon apheresis. Alternatively, Euler from the Federal Republic of Germany [14] proposed a multicenter study on plasmapheresis and subsequent pulse cyclophosphamide in severe systemic lupus erythematosus (SLE) during the 1988 World Apheresis Association Congress in Ottawa. His proposal received a high level of favourable consideration by a majority of leaders in the field of apheresis.

There are those who despite the new pharmacological concept and the negative results of the Lewis study continue to be advocates of therapeutic apheresis in the treatment of SLE. This is especially true for those patients with diffuse proliferative nephritis refractory to corticosteroids and immunosuppressives and those with major organ vasculitis secondary to SLE, or in patients with central nervous system disease.

Turning now to the area of technological progress, first some important developments in hardware will be described. A new generation of centrifuges has just entered the market. These include the BAXTER (Fenwal) CS-3000, the COBE (formerly IBM) Separa, and the FRESENIUS AS-104. All these systems provide
- improved separation properties,
- automated process control,
- fail safe operation, and
- low extracorporeal volume.

BAXTER (formerly HemaScience) also manufactures an automated system employing a rotating cylindrical membrane filter, with a membrane surface area of only 70 cm². Blood flows in a thin annular channel between the rotating membrane and stationary wall. The rotation of the filter creates shear forces and other hydrodynamic effects which virtually eliminate cellular concentration polarization and yield extraordinarily high local filtration rates. This device represents the first major advance in biomedical membrane device design since the introduction of hollow fibers 20 years ago.

This so-called Autopheresis C system was originally intended for short term, discontinuous use for plasma collection from antecubital vein. Recently, Kaplan [15] has modified the tubing system, allowing for continuous flow, double antecubital access operation. His in vivo studies have shown that the modified system is highly effective for therapeutic apheresis and provides especially high filtration fractions, i.e., high filtration rates at low values of blood flow rates.

A truly miniaturized plasma donation machine, the Ultralite, by HAEMONETICS has proved satisfactory for plasma donation and, before long, will be available in a therapeutic model.

Ongoing technical developments are driven primarily by the goal of reducing or eliminating the use of expensive and otherwise troubling albumin replacement solutions. These efforts can lower the cost of a conventional plasma exchange procedure by at least 50%. The exciting developments in

- small volume therapeutic pheresis,
- secondary filtration,
- selective precipitation, and especially
- selective or specific adsorption

should allow us, within the next few years, to replace plasma exchange in many disorders with plasma filtration and/or perfusion. This new development is likely to cause a "shake-out" among the approximately 20 companies providing or developing therapeutic apheresis systems. As a result, non-selective units may be driven from the market.

Frequent **small volume therapeutic pheresis** (SVTP) recently introduced both by Klein in the United States [16] and Gunzer in the Federal Republic of Germany [17] is performed with membrane filters of 0.1 m² active surface area. Between 500 ml and 750 ml of the patient's plasma is removed during each procedure, compared to a conventional removal volume of 2000 to 3000 ml. By increasing treatment frequency, the total plasma removal each month is comparable to conventional plasma exchange. Although simple electrolyte substitution fluids were used exclusively, patient serum albumin concentration did not decline significantly. The authors claim that the procedure is 75% less expensive than a routine plasma exchange.

Cascade filtration, introduced by Agishi in 1980 [18], likewise proposes to lower overall treatment costs by reducing or eliminating replacement fluids. Savings are realized through the use of two plasma separators with different sieving characteristics. These separators have been developed by ASAHI, BELLCO, KURARAY, TEIJIN, and TORAY and are most widely used in Japan. None of these filters can separate IgG from albumin very well and the original promise of this approach remains unrealized.

Selective **on line precipitation** for LDL removal can be accomplished by two methods. As described by Antwiler et al. [19], plasma was generated by membrane filtration and LDL precipitated with 10-35 mg% dextran sulfate in the presence of 55 mM calcium. The LDL precipitate was removed by filtration and excess calcium by dialysis. His preliminary report was based on the results of a study with four patients.

Seidel et al. [20] have subsequently introduced heparin-induced extracorporeal LDL precipitation, known by the acronym HELP, and reported on over 60 successfully treated patients with familial hypercholesterolemia resistant to conventional diet and drug therapy. A reported advantage of the HELP system over other selective LDL apheresis procedures such as immuno or chemical adsorption is the simultaneous elimination of fibrinogen.

The most important new developments are in the field of **adsorption.** In most diseases treated by apheresis, the pathogen accounts for but a small percentage of the plasma protein pool. Therefore, specific removal of the diseased protein with recovery of the patient's normal proteins is ideal. The first report dealing with on line plasma adsorption was published by Lupien in 1976 [21]. Since then, a wide variety of columns for clinical on line plasma treatment have become experimentally and commercially available. All these systems require plasma rather than whole blood as the feed and so a conventional filter must be included in the extracorporeal circuit.

Modern plasma adsorption systems such as supplied by BAXTER, EX-CORIM, and KANEKA incorporate a regeneration process utilizing two small columns. While the patient's plasma is passed through one column, the second is being regenerated using a special elution procedure. Sorption and desorption can be repeated several times without significant decrease in binding capacity. This approach overcomes the problem of low column capacity and permits virtually complete depletion of the target pathogen from the plasma pool.

Protein A, a cell wall constituent of several staphylococcal strains, is a 42,000 dalton protein with high affinity for IgG subclasses 1, 2 and 4, as well as for IgG-containing immune complexes. Two commercially available protein A columns employ protein A bound covalently to a matrix of silica in the Prosorba[R] (IMRE) column and sepharose in the EXCORIM columns.

The IMRE Prosorba column is recommended for treatment of patients with classic ITP and other thrombocytopenias, including those patients with HIV associated ITP whose platelet counts are less than 100,000/mm^3 [22]. It is also used in ongoing cancer treatment trials [23]. The exact immunological mechanism of tumor response, however, remains an issue of speculation that requires further research.

The EXCORIM Immunosorba column has been applied primarily in patients with such IgG mediated disorders as Factor VIII and IX antibodies in hemophilia [24], Goodpasture's syndrome, myasthenia gravis, and for the reduction of cytotoxic antibodies in patients awaiting renal transplantation [25]. The overall clinical results of protein A adsorption in the aforementioned conditions are promising.

ASAHI has introduced cartridges containing immobilized **amino acids** tryptophan and phenylalanine with the aim of removing autoantibodies and immune complexes. The manufacturer recommends tryptophan columns for the treatment of myasthenia gravis and chronic GBS, whereas phenylalanine is advised for acute GBS and MS. Both can be employed for SLE. Since 1983, encouraging clinical results have been published by a number of authors [26,27].

In hypercholesterolemia, sorption techniques are rapidly eclipsing traditional circuits such as plasmapheresis, cascade filtration and thermofiltration. LDL can be removed by columns containing LDL antibody, dextran sulfate or modified macroporous cellulose. The latter as yet has been investigated only in dog experiments by Behm et al. in Rostock [28]. Abundant clinical experience exists for the other two treatment modalities as reflected by numerous published articles [29,30]. Both systems are commercially available and use the two-column sorption/desorption technique. In contrast to the dextran sulfate containing Liposorber, for which single use is recommended, the highly specific LDL antibody-sepharose columns are reused for 50 procedures. Between treatments the columns are filled with a bactericidal solution and stored at 4°C.

The less specific dextran sulfate column also removes other plasma constituents. This for example applies to antithrombin III and anti-double-stranded DNA antibodies [31]. Removal of the latter could possibly prove to be adjunctive therapy in the treatment of SLE. With this system, both albumin and HDL are recovered completely as confirmed by mass balance studies of the eluted proteins. The anaphylatoxin C3a generated during the plasma separation process is fed into the adsorption device and is favourably removed during its passage through the column in both systems [32]. The aim of several ongoing trials with LDL adsorption systems is to determine whether coronary artery lesions improve.

Finally, some cutting edge technology in extracorporeal apheresis has been projected for the future. Dermatologists at Yale University [33] have introduced **extracorporeal photochemotherapy** for treatment of cutaneous T-cell lymphoma. This disease affects approximately 5 persons per million population annually. Leukapheretically obtained cells are treated with ultraviolet A light in the presence of the photoactivatable drug 8-methoxypsoralen and are then reinfused. Two treatments are carried out within a period of

4 weeks. Following this schedule, 24 of 29 erythrodermic patients in a multi-center trial achieved dramatic improvement with this therapy alone. Side effects were minimal. Such therapy may also prove to be effective against other forms of blood cancer, diabetics, and organ transplant rejection.

Further refinements of centrifugation techniques can be expected and will affect not only the recovery of cell fractions for replacement therapy but also the **removal of specific cell types** for disease modification. Filtration also may play a prominent role in the separation of cell fractions. Present filtration methods permit the removal of cells which possess the inherent property of adhering to a filter surface. It will be possible, for example, to develop filters that separate T- and B-lymphocytes by using the differentiating properties of the lymphocyte receptor sites [34].

Flow cytometry and **centrifugal elutriation** are relatively new techniques of cell sorting and cell separation that have the potential for cytoreduction and cytocollection. Although at present flow cytometry is limited in the volume of fluid that can be processed, it could become a valuable analytical tool in the preparation of solid phase columns with bound monoclonal antibodies. Such columns could affect rapid separation of large numbers of lymphocytes of given subsets, or of monocytes and other cells. Centrifugal elutriation, or counterflow centrifugation, separates cells according to differences in their sedimentation velocities and currently permits the separation of monocytes, young red blood cells, and other formed elements of the blood.

Applied ImmuneSciences, a high tech American firm from Menlo, California has packaged the various extracorporeal components into what it rather fancifully describes as an artificial lymph node ultimately targeted at prosthetic replacement of missing or deranged immune function. The company's first-generation product, currently in clinical trials, is an immune-assist device that extracts and depletes specific immune components from blood utilizing plasma separation technology. Applications for this system are in autoimmune diseases, cancer, organ transplantation, and septic shock treatment, among others. Proprietary components of the AIS technology include ICelator™ which, following apheresis, depletes plasma of selective immune complexes, and the T-Cellector™, which removes malfunctioning lymphocytes from the packed cells - before reinfusing cells together with plasma into the patient.

At a future date, this system will be complimented with a second-generation product, the **artificial lymph node**. With the help of disease-specific recombinant activators and immobilized lymphocytes, this device will enhance or suppress the immune response to a specific disease. The newly developed disease-specific proteins used in the artificial lymph node system will be supplied via technology partnerships with Chiron, Memtek and Repligen. It's far too easy to be sceptical of such futuristic concepts; but the whole history of artificial organs demonstrates that persistance and ingenuity can often confound the sceptics.

Were space to permit, LAK cell therapy [36] and other exciting developments could be added to the bouquet of new technologies in the field of apheresis.

The fertile field of future progress in this rapidly advancing and changing discipline has been shown to be obvious. There is, however, some caution that one should not be too enthusiastic about the potential of extracorporeal technology. Monocloncal antibodies and gene technology have opened wide new vistas for therapy. The recently reported recombinant human granulocyte macrophage colony stimulating factor accelerates depressed bone marrow production after high dose chemotherapy [37] and may prove that the field of sophisticated technology requiring machines may one day be eliminated.

REFERENCES

1. Abel, J.J., Rowntree, L.G., and Turner, B.B., 1914, On the removal of diffuse substances from the circulating blood of living animals by dialysis, J. Pharmacol. Exp. Ther., 5:275.
2. Abel, J.J., Rowntree, L.G., and Turner, B.B., 1914, Plasma removal with return of corpuscles (plasmapheresis), J. Pharmacol. Exp. Ther., 5:625.
3. Report of the AMA panel on therapeutic plasmapheresis. Current status of therapeutic plasmapheresis and related techniques, 1985, J. Am. med. Ass., 253:819.
4. Klein, H.G., Balow, J.E., Dau, P.C., Hamburger, M.I., Leitman, S.F., Pineda, A.A., and Tindall, R.S.A., 1986, Clinical applications of therapeutic apheresis, J. clin. Apheresis, 3:1.
5. The NIH consensus development conference on plasmapheresis in neurological diseases, 1986.
6. Rock, G., Tricklebank, G., and Members of the Canadian Apheresis Study Group, 1988, Five years of therapeutic plasma exchange in Canada, 2nd International Congress of the World Apheresis Association, Ottawa (CDN), May 18-20, 1988.
7. Dau, P. and Khatri, B.O., 1988, Double-blind study of true vs. sham plasma exchange in patients being treated with immunosuppression for acute attacks of multiple sclerosis, 2nd International Congress of the World Apheresis Association, Ottawa (CDN), May 18-20, 1988.
8. Schmitt, E. and Behm, E., 1988, Immunoadsorption vs. plasma exchange in multiple sclerosis, 2nd International Congress of the World Apheresis Association, Ottawa (CDN), May 18-20, 1988.
9. Khatri, B.O., 1988, Plasma exchange combined with immunosuppressive drug therapy in chronic progressive multiple sclerosis, 2nd International Congress of the World Apheresis Association, Ottawa (CDN), May 18-20, 1988.
10. Jayne, D.R.W, Marshall, P.D., Jones, S.J., and Lockwood, C.M., Prospective study of anti-glomerular basement membrane and anti-neutrophil cytoplasm autoantibodies in patients with a putative diagnosis of rapidly progressive glomerulonephritis and description of a subgroup with dual autoantibody positivity, Submitted for publication.
11. Clough, J., Lewis, E., Lachin, J., and the Lupus Nephritis Collaborative Study Group, 1988, A controlled trial of plasmapheresis as adjunct to conventional therapy in severe lupus nephritis. 2nd International Congress of the World Apheresis Association, Ottawa (CDN), May 18-20, 1988.
12. Austin, H.A., Klippel, J.H., and Balow, J.E., 1988, Therapy of lupus nephritis. Controlled trial of prednisone and cytotoxic drugs, New Engl. J. Med., 318:1423.
13. McCune, W.J., Golbus, J., Zelders, W., Bohlke, P., Dunne, R., and Fox, D.A., 1988, Clinical and immunologic effects of monthly administration of intravenous cyclophosphamide in severe lupus erythematosus, New Engl. J. Med., 318:1423.
14. Euler, H.H., Schroeder, J.O., Harten, P., and Löffler, H., 1988, Synchronization of plasma exchange with subsequent pulse cyclophosphamide: Induction of stable remissions in severe SLE. 2nd International Congress of the World Apheresis Association, Ottawa (CDN), May 18-20, 1988.
15. Kaplan, A.A. and Halley, S.E., 1988, Evaluation of a rotating filter for use with therapeutic plasma exchange. 34th Annual Meeting of the American Society for Artificial Internal Organs, Reno (USA), May 3-6, 1988.
16. Klein, J., Catapano, G., Feldhoff, P., Bunke, C., and Klein. E., 1988, Small volume therapeutic pheresis as an alternative to conventional pheresis. 2nd International Congress of the World Apheresis Association, Ottawa (CDN), May 18-20, 1988.
17. Gunzer, U., Klinker, E., Klink, M., Mansouri-Taleghani, B., and Günther,

C., 1988, Repeated small volume plasmapheresis in patients with immun-thrombopenia. 2nd International Congress of the World Apheresis Association, Ottawa (CDN), May 18-20, 1988.

18. Agishi, T., Kaneko, I., and Hasuo, Y., 1980, Double filtratin plasma-pheresis with no or minimal amount of blood derivate for substitution, in: Plasma exchange. Plasmapheresis - plasmaseparation, H.-G. Sieberth, ed., Schattauer, New York, p. 53-57.

19. Antiwiler, G.D., Dau, P.C., and Lobdell, D.D., 1988, Reduction of low-density lipoproteins with dextran sulfate in patients with familial hyper-cholesterolemia, J. clin. Apheresis, 4:18.

20. Seidel, D., Schuff-Werner, P., Eisenhauer, Th., Armstrong, V.W., Janning, G., Thiery, J., and Scheler, F., 1988, Long-term experience with HELP system for the treatment of severe hypercholesterolemia. 2nd International Congress of the World Apheresis Association, Ottawa (CDN), May 18-20, 1988.

21. Lupien, P.J. and Moorjani, S., 1976, A new approach to the management of familial hypercholesterolaemia: Removal of plasma-cholesterol based on the principle of affinity chromatography, Lancet, I:1261.

22. Snyder, H.W. Jr., Bertram, J., and Kiprov, D., Extracorporeal immuno-adsorption of plasma over PROSORBA Columns as treatment for idio-pathic thrombocytopenic purpura in HTLV-III infected homosexual men, In press.

23. Messerschmidt, G.L., Henry, D.H., and Snyder, H.W., 1988, Protein A immunoadsorption in the treatment of malignant disease, J. clin. Onco-logy, 6:203.

24. Nilsson, I.M., Freiburghaus, C., Sundquist, S.B., and Sandberg, H., 1984, Removal of specific antibodies from whole blood in a continuous extra-corporeal system. Plasma Ther. Transfus. Technol., 5:127.

25. Palmer, A., Taube, D., and Welsh, K., 1987, Extracorporeal immunoad-sorption of anti-HLA antibodies: Preliminary clinical experience. Trans-plant. Proc., XIX(5):3750.

26. Heininger, K., Toyka, K.V., Gaczkowski, A., Hartung, H.P., Borberg, H., and Grabensee, B., 1986, Selective removal of pathogenic factors in neurologic diseases. Plasma Ther. Transfus. Technol., 7:351.

27. Heininger, K., Gaczkowski, A., Hartung, H.P., Toyka, K.V., and Borberg, H., 1986, Plasma separation and immunoadsorption in myasthenia gravis, in: Therapeutic plasmapheresis (V), T. Oda, ed., Schattauer, Stuttgart-New York, p. 3-10.

28. Behm, E., Loth, F., and Toewe, D., 1988, A newly developed LDL-binding material. 2nd International Congress of the World Apheresis Association, Ottawa (CDN), May 18-20, 1988.

29. Busnach, G., Cappelleri, A., and Vaccarino, V., 1988, Selective and semi-selective low-density lipoprotein apheresis in familial hypercholestero-lemai, Blood Purification, 6:161.

30. Mimori, A., Takahashi, K., and Mitamura, T., 1987, Clinical evaluation of the three types of plasmapheresis in a patient with type IIa familial hypercholesterolemia, 1987, J. clin. Apheresis, 3:209.

31. Kinoshita, M., Ishikawa, H., Aotsuka, S., Yokohari, R., Funahashi, T., and Tani, N., 1988, Selective adsorption on anti-dsDNA antibodies by dextran sulfate. 2nd International Congress of the World Apheresis Asso-ciation, Ottawa, CDN, May 18-20, 1988.

32. Bosch, T., Schmidt, B., Samtleben, W., and Gurland, H.J., 1987, A new LDL-adsorption column: Ex vivo clinical performance and biocompati-bility, in: Proceedings of the 1st International Congress of the World Apheresis Association, T. Oda, Y. Shiokawa, N. Inoue, eds., ISAO Press, Cleveland, p. 576-580.

33. Heald, P.W., 1988, Extracorporeal photochemotherapy for CTCL. 2nd International Congress of the World Apheresis Association, Ottawa (CDN), May 18-20, 1988.

34. Böck, M., Krause, Ch., and Wagner, M., 1987, Transfusion of leukocyte depleted red cell concentrates and whole blood by use of a newly de-

veloped "bed-side" filter system. 5th Annual Meeting of the European Society for Haemapheresis, Cologne (FRG), September 20-23, 1987.

35. Kemshead, J.T. Heath, L., and Gibson, F.M., 1986, Magnetic microspheres and monoclonal antibodies for the depletion of neuroplastoma cells from bone marrow: Experiences, improvements and observations, Br. J. Cancer, 54:771.

36. Rosenberg, S.A., Lotze,M.T., and Muul, L.M., 1987, A progress report on the treatment of 157 patients with advanced cancer using lymphokine-activated killer cells and interleukin-2 or high dose interleukin-2 alone, New Engl. J. Med., 316:879.

37. Brandt, S., Peters, W.P., and Atwater, S.K., 1988, Effect of recombinant human granulocyte-macrophage colony-stimulating factor on hemato-poietic reconstitution after high-dose chemotherapy and autologous bone marrow transplantation, New Engl. J. Med., 318:869.

TREATMENT COMBINING PLASMAPHERESIS AND PULSE

CYCLOPHOSPHAMIDE IN SEVERE SYSTEMIC LUPUS ERYTHEMATOSUS

Johann O. Schroeder, Hans H. Euler

2nd Medical Clinic
Christian-Albrecht University Kiel
2300 Kiel 1, FRG

INTRODUCTION

The idea of curing a disease by removing harmful blood components from the patient's circulation is almost as old as human ideas about medicine[1]. With the development of devices suitable for separating plasma from the cellular blood compartments – either by continous flow centrifugation or by membrane filtration – the technical preconditions were fulfilled for applying therapeutic plasmapheresis in man. In this procedure plasma containing noxious constituents is removed and replaced by a harmless substitute.

In systemic lupus erythematosus (SLE) autoantibodies and immune complexes have been shown to play a significant role in the pathogenesis of the disease[2-4]. Since plasmapheresis has proven its ability to reduce the level of pathogenic material[5-14], conceptually it appears to be an attractive therapy for lupus[15-17]. However, to date there is no compelling evidence that this treatment modality is of therapeutic value in SLE. After initial reports demonstrating therapeutic benefit in the majority of patients receiving concomitant immunosuppressive therapy[5-7,10-14] controlled studies combining plasmapheresis with conventional immunosuppression, either in predominantly non-renal lupus[9,18] or in lupus nephritis[19], failed to substantiate a beneficial effect of plasmapheresis in the long-term course[9,18,19]. Moreover, a considerable number of patients treated with plasmapheresis alone showed an early reincrease in disease activity or even clinical deterioration[7,8,13]. This was paralleled by a rise in the levels of autoantibodies and immune complexes which – in some patients – exceeded the pretherapeutic values[7,8,13].

In view of experimental data indicating that the serum levels of specific antibodies have a negative feedback effect on the synthesis of antibodies of the same specificity[20-24], these observations may be attributed to an enhanced synthesis rate of autoantibodies induced by antibody depletion[7,13,14]. This stimulation of antibody synthesis, which is also termed "antibody rebound," has been shown in experimental studies to be related to increased B- cell proliferation[25].

This mechanism may explain the negative results of the studies performed hitherto[9,18,19]. Thus, the antibody rebound usually is regarded as detrimental to the therapeutic goal. On the other hand, it may aid in the deletion of pathogenic clones, if large doses of cytotoxic drugs are administered during the assumed period of increased proliferation, and - hence - during the period of increased vulnerability[26] of these clones. A clinical protocol that is based on these considerations should include as an essential constituent the application of high doses of an alkylating agent shortly after plasmapheresis.

We have successfully applied a protocol based on this concept of "synchronization" of plasmapheresis with pulse cyclophosphamide, in several autoantibody and immune complex-meditated diseases, such as Goodpasture's syndrome[27], pemphigus vulgaris[28] and rapidly progressive glomerulonephritis[29,30]. In SLE the first two patients treated according to this protocol achieved stable and long-lasting remissions[31]. We report here the updated results of the first eleven patients with severe SLE who were treated according to this protocol. They have now been followed up for up to three years.

PATIENT SELECTION

The admission criteria specified by the protocol included (1) a diagnosis of SLE that satisfied at least 4 American Rheumatism Association classification criteria[32], (2) clinical evidence of at least 1 clinical manifestation of active and severe lupus, such as central nervous disease, nephritis, cardiopulmonary disease, vasculitis or hematologic abnormality, (3) active disease in spite of therapy with prednisolone $\geq$ 0.5mg/kg/day and (4) informed written consent to all aspects of the protocol.

TREATMENT PROTOCOL

Before initiation of treatment, all immunosuppressive drugs such as azathioprine, cyclophosphamide or cyclosporine had to be withdrawn for at least three weeks. Plasmapheresis was performed using a hemofiltration device (Haemoprocessor 40,005; Sartorius, Göttingen, FRG) via hollow fiber membrane filters (Curesis polypropylene hollow fiber filters, Organon Teknika, BV, Turnhout, Belgium), or a centrifuge (Fenwal CS-3,000, Baxter, Deerfield, Il., USA). Each time 60 ml/kg body weight were exchanged and replaced with immunoglobulin-free 4% albumin solution. Three plasmaphereses were applied on each of days 1,2 and 3. Pulse cyclophosphamide (12 mg/kg body weight) was applied intravenously on each of days 3,4 and 5; the first infusion was given 6 hours after the third plasmapheresis. Thereafter oral cyclophosphamide was administered at an average dose of 2 mg/kg for six months. The dosage was adjusted to achieve a leukocyte count of 2,000 - 4,000/mm^3. In addition, prednisolone, which had been withdrawn for at least 3 days before the first plasmapheresis with the aim

Table 1. Clinical manifestations of the patients prior to therapy

Pat.	Age	Sex	Predominant Clinical Manifestations	ARA Criteria
L.J.	19	f	Rash, pleural effusion, pericarditis, ascites, edema, pneumonitis	5
R.S.	19	f	Rash, pleurisy, pneumonitis, weight loss (>30%), fever, thrombocytopenia	6
H.B.	26	f	Rash, arthralgia, anemia, thrombo-cytopenia, retinal hemorrhages	6
S.A.	37	f	Arthralgia, myalgia, pericarditis, headache, psychosis	5
S.D.	56	f	Seizure, arthralgia, pleural effusion, glomerulonephritis, fever	5
K.S.	18	f	Rash, pleurisy, pericarditis, membrano-proliferative GN, leukocytopenia	6
H.M.	33	f	Rash, pleurisy, pericarditis, renal insufficiency, pneumonitis, leukopenia	8
J.K.	31	f	Rash, vasculitis, digital ulcers, pericarditis, fever	6
G.M.	32	f	Rash, arthralgia, pericarditis, mesangioproliferative GN, alopecia	6
G.C.	18	f	Rash, arthralgia, fever, mesangioproliferative GN	6
S.M.	18	f	Rash, oral ulcers, fever, membrano-proliferative GN, proteinuria >25g	6

of restoring the cell proliferation capacity, was reinstituted on day 5 (initially 2 mg/kg) with subsequent tapering of the dosage to 0 during the following months.

RESULTS

Eleven female patients entered the study. The mean age was 27 (18-56) years. The mean duration of the disease at the time of entry into the study was 33 (4-81) months. The clinical manifest-ations of the 11 patients are given in Table 1. All patients suffered from multiorgan disease. In 8/11 patients the kidneys were involved. In 4 patients, renal biopsy was performed and revealed membranoproliferative (K.S, S.M) or mesangioproliferative (G.M, G.C) glomerulonephritis. In the patients with coexisting thrombocytopenia renal biopsy was not performed. All patients had been refractory to oral prednisolone; in one patient (H.B) the

application of pulse methylprednisolone (4x1,000mg/day) only
slightly reduced the symptoms of the disease. With the exception
of two patients with active glomerulonephritis (K.S., G.C.) and of
one patient whose condition deteriorated very rapidly (H.B.) all
patients had been pretreated with azathioprine (8/11), cyclophosphamide (1/11) or cyclosporine (1/11). At study entry, all
patients demonstrated high disease activity, expressed as a score
of > 20 according to the Systemic Lupus Acvity Measure[33] (SLAM).

Of the 11 patients enrolled up to January 1989 8 completed
the entire protocol. The remaining 3 patients entering the study
during the last months are currently still in the 6 months of
maintenance therapy. In one of these patients (J.K.) maintenance
therapy was prolonged to month 8 because of incompletely healed
cutaneous lesions.

In all patients the clinical condition improved rapidly. This
is demonstrated in the case of a 19-year-old patient (R.S.), who
had been admitted with severe lupus pneumonitis (s. Figure 1),
pleurisy, weight loss of more than 30%, impaired renal function,
hemolytic anemia and thrombocytopenia. Despite treatment with
prednisolone and the institution of antibiotic and antimycotic
treatment, her respiratory capacity worsened and she required
assisted ventilation. We then decided to institute the
synchronization protocol. - Six days after initiation of
treatment, the infiltrates in both lungs subsided, and they
disappeared almost completely within 16 days (s. Figure 1). Blood
urea nitrogen and creatinine fell to normal. A parallel progressive rise in hemoglobin and in the platelet count occurred.
Low levels of C4 and decreased values for the complement-mediated
inhibition of immune precipitation[34] normalized within four
weeks. The patient's weight increased by 30% and returned to

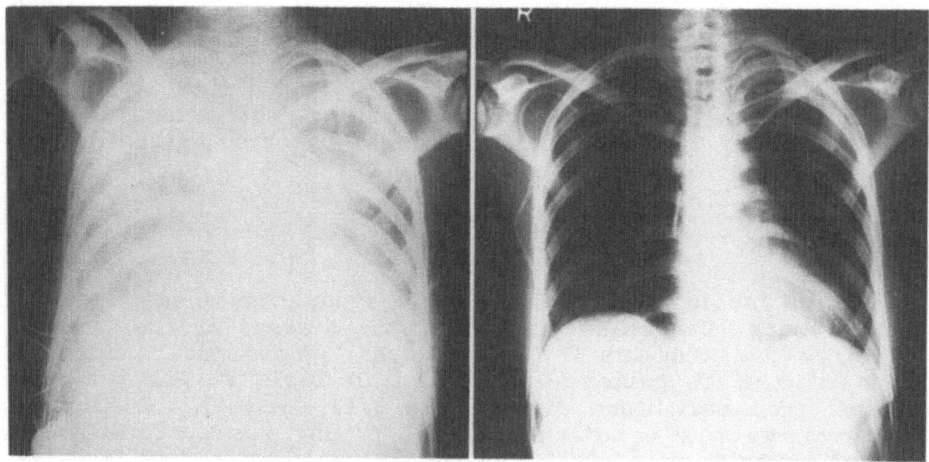

Fig 1. Chest X-ray of patient R.S., 19 years, female, 3 days
    before treatment (left side), and 16 days after initiation
    of therapy (right side).

Table 2. Clinical and laboratory parameters of patient S.R.
prior to and following therapy

R.S., 19 yrs f,		Before Therapy (3/86)	End of Therapy (9/86)	+31 Months (10/88)
Pneumonitis		++++	-	-
Polyserositis		++++	-	-
Body Weight	(kg)	38	46	60
ANA	(IgG)	1: 10,240	1: 640	1: 80
anti-ds-DNA	(%)	99	98	75
anti-ss-DNA	(%)	99	51	33
C4	(g/L)	0.07	0.46	0.38
CMIIP*	(%)	39.0	89.8	82
Hemoglobin	(g/L)	97	140	144
LDH	(U/l)	6,094	121	88
Platelets	$(10^9/l)$	35	147	244
S-Creatinine	(mg/dL)	2.9	0.7	0.5
Act. Score		35	12	0

*: Complement-mediated inhibition of immune precipitation,
determined by radioimmunoassay[34]; (normal values 82% to 100%).

normal. She was maintained on low-dose cyclophosphamide for 6
months. Then immunosuppression was withdrawn. The improvement
remained stable, and she was well without clinical signs of
disease activity at the 31-month follow-up (s. Table 2).

Similar results were obtained in the remaining ten patients.
Within the first 6 months of treatment the mean disease activity
score dropped by 22 points. In 8 patients with renal involvement a
mean pretreatment creatinine level of 2.0 mg/dL had decreased to
0.8 mg/dL at the six-month follow-up. Proteinuria >1.0 g/24h,
initially present in 7 patients, had improved from a pretreatment
mean value of 6.8 g/24h to 2.1 g/24h. All patients could be
treated as outpatients during the period of maintenance therapy.

Perhaps even more important, in the majority of patients the
clinical response remained stable after withdrawal of prednisolone
and oral cyclophosphamide. In one patient (S.A.), who complained
of fibromyalgia, prednisolone was reinstituted at month 12 at a
dosage of 10-20 mg/day. In another patient (S.D.) a complete relapse occurred at month 20, which responded to the same protocol
again after being refractory to prednisolone. 6/8 patients who
have now been followed up for 7 - 33 months (mean 21 months)
demonstrated an unchanged or even lower disease activity score up
to the last assessment point (s. Figure 2). None of these 6
patients received either corticosteroids or any immunosuppressive
agent during the posttreatment observation period (S. Figure 2).
One of these patients (H.B.) delivered a healthy child 32 months
after initiation of therapy without evidence of postpartum
reincreasing disease activity so far.

Side effects were similar in all patients. Fever and chills due to the plasmapheresis procedure were observed in 5/11 patients. Reversible alopecia and transient white blood cell depression to approx. 1.0×10^9/L at days +10 to +14 occurred in all patients. Infectious complications occurred during maintenance therapy or several months later and consisted in segmental herpes zoster in 3 patients, oral thrush in 1 patient and uncomplicated cytomegalovirus hepatitis in 2 patients. Sepsis, thrombocytopenia and hemorrhagic cystitis were not observed. In one patient (S.A.) 10 months after initiation of therapy a squamous cell carcinoma of the pharynx was diagnosed. It is very unlikely that it was related to the treatment.

DISCUSSION

This report describes the successful treatment of severely ill lupus patients with an approach that attempts to optimize the combination of plasmapheresis with an intensified immuno-suppressive regimen.

The rationale behind this approach is based on clinical and

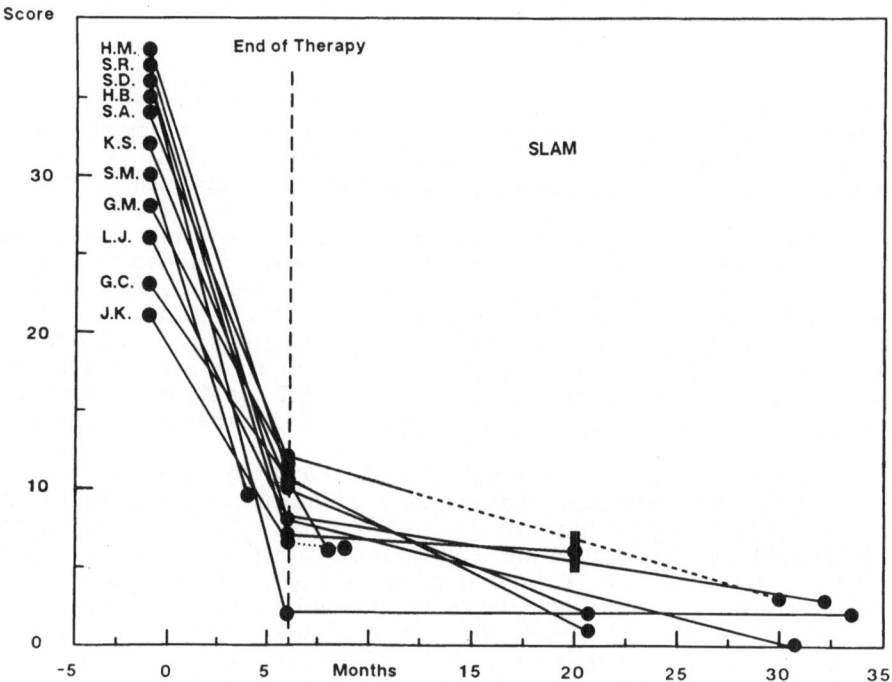

Fig 2. Activity score of all patients enrolled according to the Systemic Lupus Activity Measure (SLAM)[33]. The vertical bar designates the relapse in one patient (S.D). The dotted lines denote the reinstitution of prednisolone (- - -) in one patient (S.A) and the prolonged maintenance therapy (. . .) in one patient (J.K).

experimental data suggesting that the elimination of humoral constituents generates regulatory effects of the immune system that
compensate or overcompensate the ensuing depletion. As early as
1957 it was demonstrated that bacterial and viral antibodies
persisted at peak levels for almost two years following the administration of antigen in plasma donors who underwent biweekly
donor plasmapheresis for one year[33]. On the basis of further investigations it has been hypothesized that the humoral immune
response is provided with a mechanism by which circulating antibody itself regulates the further production of antibody of the
same specificity. It has been shown that passively administered
antibody suppresses the formation of specific antibody[20,21] and -
vice versa - that the depletion of serum antibody results in the
stimulation of new antibody synthesis that replaces and - usually
- overshoots that which has been removed[22-24]. This phenomenon has
been defined as antibody rebound. Corresponding to this, clinical
studies have shown that the elimination of autoantibodies may be
followed by increasing disease activity. This has been observed
for example in pemphigus vulgaris[36,37], in isoimmune hemolytic
anemia[38,39], in insulin-dependent diabetes mellitus in children[40]
and in myasthenia gravis[41]. In SLE, too, evidence of a serological
and clinical rebound was reported in patients treated with plasmapheresis alone[7,8,13].

The question as to how to handle this phenomenon is still
being discussed controversially. Suggestions have been made to
suppress the rebound phenomenon by maintaining immunosuppressive
drug therapy during or after plasmapheresis[42].

Contrasting to this, the schedule described in this paper
attempts to utilize the plasmapheresis-induced increase in B-cell
activity, i.e., to achieve a maximum deletion of B cell clones
considered to be involved in the pathogenesis of the disease.
Several details of the protocol were aimed at this essential
aspect of our approach: (1) no cytotoxic drugs were given before
or during plasmapheresis, to permit the restoration of B-cell
reactivity, (2) repeated large volume plasmaphereses were
performed to ensure maximum depletion of injurious plasma components, including the extravascularly distributed proportion, (3)
immunoglobulin-free substitution was used to avoid nonspecific
suppression of B-cell reactivity. Then, during the period of
assumed maximum depletion-induced B-cell activity pulse cyclophosphamide was given.

The application of this approach in the treatment of pemphigus vulgaris[28], Goodpasture's syndrome[27] and rapidly progressive
glomerulonephritis[29,30] has been shown to induce prolonged
remissions. The transfer of this approach, which also has been
termed the "stimulation-deletion model"[13] to lupus resulted in
stable remissions in the majority of cases. We observed a rapid
improvement in the disease manifestations, including recovery from
partially life-threatening situations. The beneficial effect could
be stabilized by subsequent application of low-dose cyclophosphamide. In the majority of patients we were able to withdraw all
therapy after 6 months without reoccurrence of clinical disease
activity during the follow-up period. These results, which moreover are substantiated by the remissions obtained by other groups
who applied a similar protocol[43,44,], continue to be encouraging.

However, we are aware that to date no definitive conclusions can be drawn. Since this protocol combines different treatment modalities, the weight of each constituent of the protocol is not yet clear. Obviously, the application of repeated pulses of cyclophosphamide alone has proved effective in the treatment of lupus nephritis[45] as well as in other manifestations of the disease[46]. Yet, in the former report[45] repetition of treatment was required for 18 to 48 months to maintain dialysis-free renal function. In the latter report[46] 2/9 patients had a relapse 2 to 3 months after treatment with 6 cycles of pulse cyclophosphamide. In both reports low-dose prednisone treatment was maintained after discontinuation of pulse cyclophosphamide treatment. Treatment-free long-term remissions have not been reported.

Since the central aim of this approach is the deletion of pathogenic B cell clones, the question arises whether this treatment likewise effects clones producing other than pathogenic antibodies. The desired property of an ideal approach would be the possibility to selectively destroy clones that are considered to be pathogenic[47]. This is not yet possible. However, it has been shown that the enhancement of antibody synthesis following antibody depletion is more pronounced in active clones[21,22] than in resting clones[48]. Hence, the treatment of autoantibody-mediated diseases by plasmapheresis coupled with high-dose cytotoxic drugs possibly offers a semiselective approach for the preferential deletion of active pathogenic clones. In our patients the total immunoglobulin levels returned to normal after a temporary decline, whereas the antinuclear antibodies in all patients remained distinctly below the pretherapeutic values (data not shown).

In conclusion, we regard the "synchronization" of plasmapheresis with subsequent pulse cyclophosphamide as an approach that might improve the outcome of refractory or life-threatening SLE. The question to what extent plasmapheresis contributes to the therapeutic effects of the treatment cannot be answered yet. As a first step to evaluate the role of plasmapheresis applied prior to high-dose cytotoxic drugs, a controlled study comparing repeated pulses of cyclophosphamide with and without plasmapheresis may be helpful. The design of this study and the protocol are currently being prepared by the Lupus Plasmapheresis Study Group (LPSG) constituted at the 2nd World Apheresis Association meeting in Ottawa 1988.

REFERENCES

1. H.E. Kambic and Y. Nose, "Plasmapheresis, historical perspective. Therapeutic applications and new frontiers." ISAO Press, Cleveland (1983).
2. D. Koffler, V. Agnello, R. Thoburn and H.G. Kunkel, Systemic lupus erythematosus: Prototype of immune complex nephritis in man, J Exp Med. 134:169s (1971).
3. M. Mannik, Pathophysiology of circulating immune complexes. Arthritis Rheum. 27:783 (1982).
4. J. A. Hardin, The lupus autoantigens and the pathogenesis of systemic lupus erythematosus. Arthritis Rheum. 29:457 (1986).

5. J. V. Jones, R. C. Bucknall and R. H. Cumming et al., Plasmapheresis in the management of systemic lupus erythematosus? Lancet 2: 709 (1976).

6. J. V. Jones, R. H. Cumming and P. A. Bacon et al., Evidence for a therapeutic effect of plasmapheresis in patients with systemic lupus erythematosus. Q J Med. 48:555 (1979).

7. J. V. Jones, M. F. Robinson, R. K. Parciany, L. F. Layfer and B. McLeod, Therapeutic plasmapheresis in systemic lupus erythematosus. Arthritis Rheum. 24:1113 (1981).

8. R. Schlansky, R. J. Dehoratius, T. Pincus and K. S. K. Tung, Plasmapheresis in systemic lupus erythematosus. A cautionary note. Arthritis Rheum. 24:49 (1981).

9. N. Wei, J. H. Klippel and D. P. Huston et al., Randomised trial of plasma exchange in mild systemic lupus erythematosus. Lancet 1: 17 (1983).

10. H. F. Parry, L. J. Nineham and C. J. Moran et al., Plasma exchange in systemic lupus erythematosus. Ann Rheum Dis. 40:224 (1981).

11. L. Kater, R.H.W.M. Derksen and F. A. Houwert et al., Effect of plasmapheresis in active systemic lupus erythematosus. Neth J Med. 24: 209 (1981).

12. C. M. Lockwood, S. Worlledge, A. Nicholas, C. Cotton and D. K. Peters, Reversal of impaired splenic function in patients with nephritis or vasculitis (or both) by plasma exchange. N Engl J Med. 300:524 (1979).

13. J. V. Jones, Plasmapheresis in SLE. Clin Rheum Dis. 8:243 (1982).

14. J. D. Clough and L. H. Calabrese, Theoretical aspects of immune complex removal by plasmapheresis. Plasma Ther Transfus Technol. 2: 73 (1981).

15. American Society of Apheresis, Clinical applications of therapeutic apheresis. Report of the Clinical Applications Committee. J Clin Apheresis. 3:30 (1986).

16. K. H. Shumak and G. A. Rock, Therapeutic plasma exchange. N Engl J Med. 310: 762 (1984).

17. J. V. Jones, J. D. Clough, J. R. Klinenberg and P. Davis, The role of plasmapheresis in the rheumatic diseases. J Lab Clin Clin Med. 97:589 (1981).

18. French Cooperative Study Group, A randomised trial of plasma exchange in severe acute systemic lupus erythematosus: Methodology and interim analysis. Plasma Ther Trans Tech. 6:535 (1985).

19. J. Clough, E. Lewis, J. Lachin and the Lupus Nephritis Collaborative Study Group, A controlled trial of plasmapheresis as adjunct to conventional therapy in severe lupus nephritis. Abstr. WAA, 2: 2-1 (1988).

20. J. W. Uhr and J. B. Baumann, Antibody formation. I. Suppression of antibody formation by passively administered antibody. J Exp Med. 113:935 (1961).

21. H. Chang, S. Schneck, N. I. Brody, A. Deutsch and G. W. Siskind, Studies on the mechanism of the suppression of active antibody synthesis by passively administered antibody. J Immunol. 102:37 (1969).

22. M. W. Graf and J.W. Uhr, Regulation of antibody formation by serum antibody, I. Removal of specific antibody by means of immunoadsorption, J Exp Med. 131:1175 (1069).

23. J.-C. Bystryn, M. W.Graf, J. W. Uhr, Regulation of antibody formation by serum antibody. II. Removal of specific antibody by means of exchange transfusion. J Exp Med. 132:1279 (1970).

24. J.-C. Bystryn, I. Schenkein and J. W. Uhr, A model for the regulation of antibody synthesis by serum antibody. Prog Immunol. 1:627 (1971).

25. B. C. Sturgill, and M. J. Worzniak, Stimulation of proliferation of 19S antibody-forming cells in the spleens of immunized guinea-pigs after exchange transfusion. Nature 228: 1304 (1970).

26. W. R. Bruce, B. E. Meeker and F. A. Valeriote, Comparison of the sensitivity of normal hematopoietic and transplanted lymphoma colony-forming cells to chemotherapeutic agents administered in vivo. J Natl Cancer Inst. 37:223 (1966).

27. H. H. Euler, L. Kleine, H. J. Gutschmidt and J. D. Herrlinger, Effect of early plasmapheresis and high-dose cyclophosphamide therapy in Goodpasture's syndrome, in: " Plasmapheresis in Immunology and Oncology" , J. H. Beyer, H. Borberg, C. Fuchs and G. A. Nagel eds., S. Karger, Basel (1982).

28. H. H. Euler, H. Löffler and E. Christophers, Synchronization of plasmapheresis and puls cyclophosphamide in pemphigus vulgaris. Arch Dermatol. 123: 1205 (1987).

29. H. H. Euler, U. Krey, H. J. Gutschmidt and H. Löffler, Partial synchronization of plasmapheresis and immunosuppression in autoimmune diseases: Experimental and clinical results, in: "Therapeutic plasmapheresis: A critical look", Y. Nosé, P. S. Malchesky and J. W. Smith eds., ISAO Press, Cleveland (1984).

30. H.-J. Gutschmidt, H. H. Euler, J. Albrecht, F. Asbeck, L.H. Kleine, C.v. Klinggräff and H. Löffler, Cyclophosphamide stoss-therapy synchronized with plasmapheresis in rapidly progressive glomerulonephritis, Dtsch med Wschr. 111:1439 (1986).

31. J. O. Schröder, H. H. Euler and H. Löffler, Synchronization of plasmapheresis and pulse cyclophosphamide in severe lupus erythematosus. Ann Int Med. 107: 344 (1987).

32. E. M. Tan, A. S. Cohen and J. F. Fries et al., The 1982 revised criteria for the classification of systemic lupus erythematosus. Arthritis Rheum. 25:1271 (1982).

33. M. H. Liang, S. Stern and J. M. Esdaile, Towards an operational definition of SLE activity for clinical research. Clin Rheum Dis. in press (1989).

34. J. A. Schifferli, S. R. Bartolotti and D. K. Peters, Inhibition of immune precipitation by complement. Clin exp Immunol. 42:387 (1980).

35. J. Smolens, J. Stokes and A.B. Vogt, Human plasmapheresis and its effects on antibodies, J Immunol. 79:434 (1957).

36. J. C. Roujeau, C. Andre, J. Revuz and R. Touraine, Effects of various immunosuppressive regimens on the "Rebound phenomenon" induced by plasma exchange in pemphigus, in: "Plasmapheresis. Therapeutic Applications and New Techniques", Y. Nosé, P. S. Malchesky, J. W. Smith and R. S. Krakauer eds., Raven Press, New York (1983).

37. J. C. Guillaume, J. C. Roujeau and P. Morel et al., Controlled study of plasma exchange in pemphigus, Arch Dermatol. 124:1659 (1988).

38. G. R. Barclay, M. Ayoub Greiss and S. J. Urbaniak, Adverse effect of plasma exchange on anti-D production in rhesus immunisation owing to removal of inhibitory factors. Br Med J. 280: 1569 (1980).
39. J. P. Isbister, A. Ting and K. M. Seeto, Development of Rh-specific maternal autoantibodies following intensive plasmapheresis for Rh immunisation during pregnancy. Vox Sang. 33:353 (1977).
40. J. Ludvigsson, L. Heding and G. Lieden et al., Plasmapheresis in the initial treatment of insulin-dependent diabetes mellitus in children. Br Med J. 286:176 (1983).
41. J. Newsom-Davis, S. G. Wilson, A. Vincent and C. D. Ward, Long-term effects of repeated plasma exchange in myasthenia gravis. Lancet I: 464, (1979).
42. Council on Scientific Affairs, Council Report, Current status of plasmapheresis and related techniques, Report of the AMA panel on therapeutic plasmapheresis, JAMA 253:819 (1985)
43. W. G. Barr , E. A. Hubbell and J. A. Robinson, Persistently active lupus erythematosus treated with intermittent plasmapheresis and bolus cyclophosphamide, in: "Proceedings of the first international congress of the world apheresis association: Therapeutic Plasmapheresis VI" T. Oda, Y. Shiokawa, N. Inoue, eds., ISAO-Press, Cleveland, (1987).
44. C. C. Zielinski, C. Müller and J. S. Smolen, A controlled study on the treatment of severe active systemic lupus erythematosus by plasmapheresis, in: EULAR Symposium Vienna, Abstr. 88 (1985).
45. H. A. Austin, J. H. Klippel and J. E. Balow et al., Therapy of lupus nephritis. Controlled trial of prednisone and cytotoxic drugs. N Engl J Med. 314: 614 (1986).
46. W. J. McCune, J. Golbus, W. Zeldes, P. Bohlke, R. Dunne and D. A. Fox, Clinical and immunologic effects of monthly administration of intravenous cyclophosphamide in severe systemic lupus erythematosus. N Engl J Med. 318: 1423 (1988).
47. J. C. Bystryn, Editorial: Plasmapheresis Therapy of Pemphigus, Arch Dermatol. 124:1702 (1988)
48. R.H. W. Derksen, H.J. Schuurman, and F.H.J. Gmelig Meyling et al., Rebound and overshoot after plasma exchange in humans, J Lab Clin Med. 104:35 (1984).

INDEX